What people are sa

Living Beyond Lyme

Living Beyond Lyme is an excellent addition to the Lyme disease library of those who have tick-borne illness in their families, as well as the doctors and mental health practitioners from whom these patients seek help. Dr. Trunzo's extensive knowledge of Lyme disease and ACT (Acceptance & Commitment Therapy) provided the foundation upon which he developed a new and effective model for working with those who are suffering. I applaud him for the fine job he has done explaining this complex illness, and how ACT can help those who are attempting to cope with the functional issues that produce a second source of trauma for these patients.
Sandy Berenbaum, LCSW, co-author: *When Your Child Has Lyme Disease: A Parent's Survival Guide*

Living Beyond Lyme is a much-needed and extremely welcome book addressing a specific approach to helping those with chronic Lyme disease manage the psychological and interpersonal effects of this life-altering illness.

Falling ill with chronic Lyme disease is very often a true medical nightmare. It is more typical than not for sufferers to be ping-ponged between a myriad of medical specialists before ever being given a proper diagnosis. Once diagnosed, which can take place years and even decades after the first symptoms appear, chronic Lyme sufferers are then plunged down the rabbit hole of medical treatment which is definitely not for the faint of heart.

All this to say that being struck by this multi-system, neurological, immunosuppressive illness often causes sufferers no end of psychological and emotional struggles and requires a complete paradigm shift about many things including: being repeatedly] in which friends and family may or may not 'show up' as needed; as well as the sufferer having no option but to dig deep to find their own wellspring of strength and resilience which is an absolute requirement for them to go the distance in their healing journey.

In order to cope with this chronic illness, Lyme sufferers require a psychological framework that will help them address the myriad of symptoms that they must endure from moment to moment, hour to hour, day to day, as well as the loneliness, fear and isolation that Lyme disease often creates.

In *Living Beyond Lyme*, author Joseph Trunzo, PhD, has provided us with a very important psychological framework which teaches mindfulness skills and a values-based understanding in order to help sufferers create a more integrated, accepting and supportive approach to co-existing and living more amicably with the daily pain and challenges of chronic Lyme disease.

Lori Dennis, MA, Registered Psychotherapist, and author of *Lyme Madness: Rescuing My Son Down the Rabbit Hole of Chronic Lyme Disease*

Living Beyond Lyme

Reclaim Your Life From Lyme Disease
and Chronic Illness

Living Beyond Lyme

Reclaim Your Life From Lyme Disease and Chronic Illness

Joseph J. Trunzo

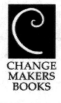

CHANGE
MAKERS
BOOKS

Winchester, UK
Washington, USA

First published by Changemakers Books, 2018
Changemakers Books is an imprint of John Hunt Publishing Ltd., No. 3 East Street,
Alresford, Hampshire SO24 9EE, UK
office1@jhpbooks.net
www.johnhuntpublishing.com
www.changemakers-books.com

For distributor details and how to order please visit the 'Ordering' section on our website.

Text copyright: Joseph J. Trunzo 2017

ISBN: 978 1 78535 041 2
978 1 78535 042 9 (ebook)
Library of Congress Control Number: 2017946209

All rights reserved. Except for brief quotations in critical articles or reviews, no part of this book may be reproduced in any manner without prior written permission from the publishers.

The rights of Joseph J. Trunzo as author have been asserted in accordance with the Copyright, Designs and Patents Act 1988.

A CIP catalogue record for this book is available from the British Library.

Design: Stuart Davies

Printed and bound by CPI Group (UK) Ltd, Croydon, CR0 4YY, UK

We operate a distinctive and ethical publishing philosophy in all areas of our business, from our global network of authors to production and worldwide distribution.

Contents

Acknowledgments   xiv
Introduction   1

Chapter 1 — The Lyme Trap   6
You're Not Alone in the Lyme Trap
The Lyme Trap in Action: Diane
Lyme Disease: Controversies and Confusion
Transmission of Lyme
How Common Is Lyme?
Symptom Presentation
Lyme Disease and Psychiatric Symptoms
Pay Attention to Your Mental Health
What Can You Do for Your Health?
Lyme-Driven Psychiatric Symptoms Case Example: Eddie
Eddie's Diagnosis
Treating Lyme Symptoms
IDSA and ILADS
Conflict in Practice
ACT and the Lyme Trap
Taking Control Where You Can: ACT in Action
Transform Your Suffering, No Matter the Cause

Chapter 2 — Acceptance and Commitment Therapy   26
ACT: What's It All About?
The History of ACT
Psychological Flexibility
Being Open
Defusion
Acceptance
Being Centered
Self-As-Context

Contact with the Present Moment
Being Engaged
Values
Committed Action
The Hexaflex
Psychological Inflexibility
A Return to Mindfulness
Mindfulness Exercise: Mindful Senses
Psychological Flexibility and Lyme

Chapter 3 — Don't Believe Everything You Think　　　**44**
The Importance of Defusion
Your Thinking Self
Your Observing Self
Right or Wrong, It Doesn't Matter
Easier Said Than Done?
ACT in Metaphors and Exercises
The Basics
Your Thoughts Are Like a Menu — Pick the One You Want
Getting Hooked
Passengers on the Bus
The "Silly" Ones
The Mindful Ones
The Experiential Ones
A Mindfulness Defusion Exercise: Dandelions in the Wind
Boat on the Water
Caveats and Pitfalls

Chapter 4 — The Paradox of Acceptance　　　**63**
What Is Acceptance?
Common Misunderstanding about Acceptance
Acceptance in ACT
Non-Chronic Illness Case Example: Emily
Emily and Experiential Avoidance

Acceptance versus Experiential Avoidance
Take a Ride on a Balloon
Climbing Mountains
The Reward of Acceptance
Acceptance in Chronic Illness: Choice versus Control
We Are Problem-Solving Machines
Chronic Illness + Problem Solving = Experiential Avoidance
A Different Path: Acceptance
Why Acceptance Seems Counterintuitive
Acceptance in Action
Acceptance and Willingness Exercise: Giving It Form
Moving Forward with Acceptance
Lyme and Chronic Illness: Unwanted Guests at the Party of Your Life
Lessons from Paralysis to Overcome Paralysis
We Are Always Whole

Chapter 5 — You Are When You Are: Self-As-Context　　83
Getting Centered
Perspective Taking
The Lighthouse
Self-Stories
Noticing
Be Here Now, Not There Then
Case Example: Jennifer
Self-As-Context in Lyme and Chronic Illness
I Don't Have Any Negative Self-Stories
My Life Was Better Before I Got Sick
Case Example: Rebecca
Defusion and Acceptance in Self-As-Context
Let's Watch a Game of Chess
Conclusions

Chapter 6 — Contact with the Present Moment   100
Staying Rooted in the Moment
It's a Skill, Not a Gift
Case Examples
It's Not Just You
The Basics
Noticing
Being Present versus Past or Future
Using Anchors
Mindfulness and Lyme
The Detective and the Documentarian
Conclusions

Chapter 7 — What Matters Most?   113
Leading a Values-Driven Life
Values in ACT
Values Are Freely Chosen
Values Are Action Based
Values Are Intrinsic
Values Are Not Goals
Values Are Big Picture and Unifying
Want to Find Your Values? Look to Your Pain
Dealing with Values Conflicts
Values in Lyme and Chronic Illness
Case Example: Megan
Values in Lyme
Values Exercises
Conclusions

Chapter 8 — Doing Is Living: Committed Action   134
It's Called ACT for a Reason
You Own It, so Own Up to It
The Power and Pitfalls of Choice
The Myth of Motivation

Case Example: John
I Promise, It Will Hurt (but not all of the time)
Goal-Directed Action versus Value-Directed Action
Barriers
Willingness
Committed Action and Chronic Illness
Megan Revisited
The Tradition of Behavior Therapy
Conclusions

Chapter 9 — Bringing It All Together 150
Some Final Thoughts
The Hexaflex Revisited
Isolation Is the Enemy, Connection Is the Cure
Future Directions
My Hope for You

From the Author 158
Further Reading 159
Bibliography 161

To all who suffer from the ravages of Lyme disease or any devastating illness. Your courage in the face of adversity inspires the work that follows.

Acknowledgments

As anyone who's ever written a book knows, it's not something that can be done in isolation. It's impossible to list all of the people who have contributed, in one way or another, to this project. As such, if I miss anyone, please accept my apology and know that you are appreciated.

I cannot adequately express my gratitude to Julie Luongo, one of my oldest and dearest friends, for her guidance in shaping the idea for this book, her editorial expertise, constructive feedback, and steadfast honesty and support. I also want to thank Timothy Ward, my publisher from Changemakers Books, for understanding and embracing my vision for this project. He took a chance on a first-time author and has been a tremendous support and guide through this process. I am eternally grateful. Likewise, the staff at Changemakers Books and John Hunt Publishing have been wonderful. They're a professional and supportive group of people who've made this process manageable and have immeasurably improved the finished product. Also, a special thanks to Jon Whitbeck for his help in selecting the cover art, creating LivingBeyondLyme.com, and crafting the social media presence for the book.

A number of people read early versions of this manuscript and provided me with invaluable feedback. These include Drs. Deborah Sepinwall, Rebecca Zisserson, Dina Habboushe, Carolynn Kohn, and Rima Saad. Thank you for your time, expertise, feedback, and friendship. I also want to thank my colleagues in the Applied Psychology Department and the College of Arts and Sciences at Bryant University for their overall support, encouragement, and patience regarding my work on this project. Without the support of the University (especially the Faculty and Staff Writing Retreats), I never would have found the time to write this book.

Acknowledgments

Broadly, I am grateful to those who have invested their time and energy in my training as a psychologist. To all of my mentors, supervisors, and peers, I am humbled by your talent and generosity. Specifically, I want to thank the ACT community for their openness, willingness to share ideas, and dedication to continually improving the overall ACT approach. I especially want to thank Steve Hayes for his encouragement in moving forward with this project. Both he and Russ Harris were generous in their permission to include versions of many of their techniques and exercises in this book.

I am also grateful to my colleagues in the Lyme community, who have always been welcoming to me and supportive of my efforts to do work in this area. They are a wonderful group of people and I have unending respect for them.

To all of my clients, thank you for sharing your deepest selves with me and giving me the honor of working with you to improve your lives. I learn from you every day and am better for the time we spend together.

Last, but certainly not least, I owe an unpayable debt of gratitude to my family. To my parents, Tony and Karen, for their unwavering support of my professional and personal values and goals. Without their foundation, nothing good in my life would have ever happened. To my loyal canine companions, Gracie and Bear, for lying quietly at my feet over many hours of writing, providing comfort and joy in difficult moments. And finally, to my wife Melissa, whose advice and guidance on this project has been invaluable from day one, and to my daughters, Rhiannon and Lily, who are the pure joys of my life. They all sacrificed more than anyone for this project, and I love them all the more for it. They gave up time with their husband and father and never complained about it or questioned the importance of the work. In fact, they were openly excited and proud, which kept me going more times than I can count. This did not go unnoticed. I hope the finished product is worthy of their support and sacrifice.

Introduction

If you're reading this book, chances are that you are suffering. *Living Beyond Lyme* is all about finding a way to redefine your emotional and physical pain so you can live your life in a rich, vital, and meaningful way while you overcome seemingly insurmountable obstacles regarding your health. In the following pages, I will give you practical tools that have the potential to transform your present experience and ultimately your life. I've seen time and again the scientifically supported psychological approach, called ACT, have powerful and profound effects on my clients, and I'm hopeful that they will help you. Before we begin, however, there are several points that are important for you to keep in mind as we move forward on this journey together.

This book is designed to help readers improve functioning and quality of life while on the journey to getting well. That said, as you will see, the symptom profile for Lyme disease is remarkably similar to a number of other illnesses—so much so that Lyme has often been called "The Great Imitator" because it can look like so many other things—Multiple Sclerosis, Chronic Fatigue Syndrome, Fibromyalgia, depression, and anxiety, just to name a few. While *Living Beyond Lyme* is geared towards people with Lyme disease, it is my sincere wish that people with other chronic illnesses will use the approaches described in this book to improve their lives or the lives of those they love. I hope that those treating people with Lyme or chronic illness—psychologists, therapists, social workers, physicians, nurses—will find it useful in their work as well. The ACT approach can help anyone develop more psychological flexibility and weather any of the storms of life with more resilience.

In terms of how best to read this book, I would recommend reading it in order, at least once. After you've gotten the full picture of the ACT model, feel free to jump around and re-read parts that you think might be useful in the moment. There are multiple exercises throughout the book that, if you find them to be helpful, you can refer to as frequently as you like. While I recognize that many people will simply read the exercises and will not actually do them, I still want to encourage you to engage as much as you can. You can probably get something out of just reading them, but ACT is fundamentally an approach of *doing*. The more you do, the more you'll get out of it.

Some books are meant to be read, others are meant to be experienced, and the book in your hands is the latter. I don't think reading it as quickly as you can will give you the most you can get out of it, so take your time, read, re-read, savor, and experience it. I wrote this book from a place of compassion, and I hope that shows in obvious ways. But turning it over in your head and your heart a few times might help you connect with that intention.

I also ask that you read this book with patience and an open mind. The ACT model is a bit paradoxical. It challenges preconceived notions and presents some ideas and approaches that may feel unfamiliar or unexpected to you at first. Please, read on and see where it goes. You might be pleasantly surprised at where you end up.

What should you expect to get out of reading this book? Well, I hope it's nothing short of a transformative experience that sets you on the path of leading a rich, vital, and meaningful life while you work towards wellness. These are big expectations of course. My own experience with these kinds of books is that while I may not find *everything* in them to be of use, I almost always find *something* in them that is. Even if that's the most you get out of reading *Living Beyond Lyme*, I will have, in some small way, done my job.

It is critically important to understand that this is not a "Lyme Cure" book. I'm not a medical doctor, so I can't write that book.

There are, however, many books on the market that deal with curing this illness, and I strongly encourage you to read the ones that may be useful to you. Unfortunately, despite everyone's best efforts, many people experience longer-term symptoms of Lyme. Even in its acute phase, it could take weeks or months for Lyme symptoms to remit. If Lyme becomes chronic, symptoms can linger for extended periods of time, dramatically affecting your life. In other words, even as you're working at curing your Lyme, there will inevitably be a period of time where it is profoundly affecting your ability to live the life you want to live. Reading books focused on curing your illness may be essential to improving your health and wellness, but they often do not address the fundamental issue of how to deal with your immediate difficulties. This leaves you in the position of waiting for your illness to be cured instead of living your life. This is the precise issue *Living Beyond Lyme* was designed to address.

As you may or may not know, Lyme disease has a complex medical-political history that is quite controversial. Many people who are regarded as experts in treating Lyme disease would bristle at the very title of this book, which characterizes Lyme as a chronic disease. In no way do I thoroughly address these issues. While I discuss them in Chapter 1 in a very "this is what you need to know" sort of way, there are well-investigated, comprehensively written books that cover this topic in great depth. You should read them (there is a recommended reading list at the end of the book). However, I don't believe that adding to this conversation is absolutely necessary to helping you live well right now.

The diagnosis of Lyme disease can be a very tricky and convoluted process, making you feel like you're on the worst possible roller-coaster ride. Is it Lyme? MS? Chronic Fatigue? Depression? Medicine may not have answered those questions for you yet. But you don't need them in order for this book to be helpful to you. What's NOT in question is that things aren't how you want them to be and that you're suffering. The purpose of this book is to help you reclaim your life—*right now*—regardless of what may be happening with your illness.

Much of what's in this book is built on material generated by the scientists who founded ACT. I put my own spin on things and tailor the approach for people dealing with Lyme, but almost everything I share with you has its roots in other people's work. Turn to the back of the book and look at the extensive reference list. It's there for a reason. I am standing on the shoulders of proverbial giants here, and I am eternally grateful to them (see the Acknowledgments).

ACT is a relatively new therapeutic approach in the behavioral sciences, but it's grounded in solid scientific research and has been developed by top-notch behavioral scientists. While the ACT model has solid scientific merit, its use in a Lyme disease population has not been scientifically studied. The content of this book is based on my clinical experience using a scientifically based treatment approach in a specific population. It is my sincere hope that this work serves as a springboard to doing the scientific work needed in this area.

If you find the tools presented here to be helpful to you, please seek out the extensive ACT resources available and expand your knowledge of this approach to living your life. While I didn't create ACT, I have been trained in it, I use it with my clients, and I try my best to practice and use it in my own life. Like most people, I'm not always successful in this endeavor, but that's okay. I encourage you to be gentle with yourself on this front. Change doesn't always come easily.

As a psychologist who knows a good bit about two worlds, the world of ACT and the world of Lyme disease, I think ACT has a lot to offer people who are suffering from Lyme and other chronic illnesses and vice versa. This book is my attempt to introduce these two worlds to one another. I believe that good things will come of it for everyone. My hope is that in the process,

Introduction

you will experience something transformative. You deserve to live a rich, fulfilling, meaningful life *right now* in this moment—today, tomorrow, and for the rest of your life—regardless of Lyme disease or any other illness. It is my sincere belief that what follows in the pages of this book will help you do this, to reclaim your life, and set you on a path to Living Beyond Lyme.

If you are interested in participating in a research project regarding your experience of this book, please go to LivingBeyondLyme.com and click on the "Research" link. Thank you!

Chapter 1

The Lyme Trap

When life kicks you, let it kick you forward.
Kay Yow

You're Not Alone in the Lyme Trap
If you've had to manage chronic symptoms of Lyme disease, you understand the title of this chapter perfectly. There are hundreds of thousands of people worldwide stuck in the Lyme Trap—working to get well and trying to live a meaningful life despite having a debilitating disease that robs them of everything they hold dear. For these people, Lyme leads to untold pain, loss, and suffering—with little consensus from the medical community on how best to help. The purpose of this book is to show you how Acceptance and Commitment Therapy (ACT, said as one word) can help you escape the Lyme Trap and lead a richer, more vital, and more meaningful life while you're on your journey to wellness.

Lyme is a tricky disease that's surrounded by controversy in all facets of the illness—transmission, diagnosis, and treatment. You may be all too familiar with these issues already, but it's worth reviewing them for newcomers, professionals, caregivers, and family members. This chapter alone could be an entire book (several books in fact), but I'll do my best to present the most important information in a clear, concise, and unbiased way. I strongly encourage you to educate yourself about this disease as much as possible. I have included a list of excellent resources later in the book to help you do this. However, in the spirit of escaping the Lyme Trap, this chapter will give you a sufficient overview.

Because the medical and political aspects of this illness are incredibly complex, the best way to understand them is often through case examples. The case of Diane illustrates why Lyme can be so difficult to cope with, diagnose, and treat.

The Lyme Trap in Action: Diane

Diane is a 34-year-old woman who has worked in an advertising agency since she graduated from college 12 years ago. She is married and has two children, a 4-year-old daughter and 2-year-old son. Diane was an energetic, intelligent woman who was highly valued for her skills by her employer. She had a wide network of friends and was close to her family. She loved to hike, camp, bike, run, and spend time outdoors. She was fit, healthy, and had no history of any medical or mental health problems. She was, for all intents and purposes, perfectly healthy and quite happy with her life.

Like any mother of two young children, she was often tired by the end of the day. However, she noticed that her fatigue was worsening. She became increasingly tired earlier in the day, often to the point of almost falling asleep at her job. She struggled to maintain her regular exercise routine. Where she used to run 3 miles without a problem, just walking around the block became a painful chore for her. Her thinking was clouded. She had difficulty finding words, couldn't concentrate, and her creativity had all but abandoned her. She was feeling soreness and pain in her joints and often had tingling sensations in her limbs, hands, and feet. She felt irritable, despondent, and anxious, sometimes having full-blown panic attacks that would last for extended periods of time.

Diane finally sought the advice of her primary care physician with whom she had a long and trusting relationship. Her doctor ran all of the usual blood tests, including a Lyme test, all of which came back negative. Her doctor could not seem to find any evidence of a medical cause for her symptoms. She sent Diane to a series of specialists, including an infectious disease doctor, all of whom ran additional tests. None found any medical reason for her symptoms.

Diane grew increasingly frustrated. She was forced to take a medical leave of absence from her job and wasn't sure when—or if—she would return. She was less and less able to be involved in the day-to-day care and activities of her children. These responsibilities fell more and more to her husband who was feeling distressed and overburdened. Diane and her husband began fighting frequently, a dynamic that had never really existed in their relationship before her illness.

Finally, Diane's doctor suggested that some of her symptoms might be psychiatrically based and referred her to a psychiatrist and a therapist, both of whom diagnosed Diane with major depression. The psychiatrist prescribed antidepressant medications and the therapist worked hard with Diane to improve her symptoms, but she did not experience any real progress or feel any better.

She and her husband began researching her symptoms and were coming to believe that, despite her negative lab work, Lyme disease might be at the root of her problems. She raised this issue with her primary care and infectious disease doctors, both of whom informed her that because she tested negative for Lyme, that simply couldn't be the problem. When Diane questioned the accuracy of the tests, she was referred back to her psychiatrist. But Diane felt strongly that her symptoms were not psychiatrically based.

Further research on Diane's part uncovered the existence of a controversy in medicine about the diagnosis and treatment of Lyme disease. Apparently, some doctors believed current testing methods to be inadequate. Moreover, they claimed that some instances of the disease could be chronic in nature, often requiring long-term high doses of antibiotics, sometimes intravenously, for adequate treatment. This was in direct contrast to the established guidelines for the treatment of Lyme, which were being followed by her medical providers.

Diane was at a loss. She was receiving one set of advice from her current doctors that seemed contradictory to what some other doctors would recommend. She wanted to seek advice from some of these other Lyme specialists, but their waiting lists were very long, *most of them did not take insurance, and their fees were often very expensive. Money had been tight since her medical leave, and she could not afford to see one of these doctors for a second opinion.*

In the midst of all of this, Diane's symptoms continued to get worse, not better, and she was experiencing unpleasant side effects from the psychiatric medications she was taking. She didn't know what to do or where to turn. It seemed as though everyone who was treating her had the best of intentions, but she simply wasn't getting better and couldn't afford the possibility of other treatment.

Diane was stuck in the Lyme Trap.

Lyme Disease: Controversies and Confusion

Diane's case may seem extreme, but unfortunately it is all too common. She is very much caught in the Lyme Trap—unable to get the treatment she may need and feeling unable to live her life until she gets well. The division in medicine regarding this illness is a significant contributing factor to Diane's circumstance. While it's possible that her symptoms are psychiatrically based, there are factors that are inconsistent with this diagnosis (lack of history, no triggering events). Moreover, as any responsible behavioral health professional would tell you, always rule out medical causes for psychological problems first. Diane tested negative for Lyme disease, so why would any reasonable health professional advocate pursuit of further treatment for an illness she did not have? If doctors agreed to every patient request based on what was read online, health care costs would skyrocket even higher than they have already. Yet, there are respected medical professionals who question the accuracy of the testing used and the conclusions Diane's doctors have reached. Who does she believe? What should she do?

There are no easy answers to these questions. Clearly, there are multiple medical, scientific, and political factors that affect the diagnosis and treatment of this illness. It's not the purpose of this chapter to argue one point versus the other, nor is it my intention to convince you of any particular point of view. My goal is to simply put forth factual information to highlight the overall problem. You need to decide what the best course of action is in *your* particular circumstance. This can be hard, but I'll talk a lot more about how best to make decisions later in the book. For now, let's cover the basics and begin building the foundation for escaping the Lyme Trap.

Transmission of Lyme

People contract Lyme disease when they are bitten by ticks that carry the Lyme bacteria, technically referred to as *Borrelia burgdorferi* (*B. burgdorferi*), named after Willy Burgdorfer, who discovered the bacteria in 1982 (Burgdorfer, 1993). Ticks are a type of arachnid, and they feed on the blood of small and large mammals, such as mice, squirrels, other rodents, and of course deer and people. As ticks attach themselves to these animals, they can both pick up and transmit *B. burgdorferi* through the blood of the host (Embers et al, 2013). There are many types of ticks, but Lyme is mostly associated with the deer tick. There is some debate as to whether or not other types of ticks, such as dog ticks, transmit the infection. But most scientific research indicates that deer ticks are the primary mode of disease transmission (Piesman and Happ, 1997; Magnarelli and Anderson, 1988). There are many questions about whether or not transmission can also occur via other means, such as sexual contact, childbirth, and mosquito bites to name a few, but the scientific studies to support these concerns are limited or non-existent.

Regardless, once the bacteria enter the bloodstream, they start to do considerable biological damage. *B. burgdorferi* is what's known as a spirochete. The bacteria have a corkscrew shape that allows them to bore into the cells of the body, disrupt the functioning of those cells, and cause the symptoms of Lyme that can be so devastating. *B. burgdorferi* does not discriminate against what kinds of cells it will invade. It often settles in the joints but can also infect organ tissue, other soft tissue, and the nervous system. This is what accounts for the wide range of symptoms one might experience with this illness, earning Lyme the moniker "The Great Imitator" (Pachner, 1989; Burdash and Fernandes, 1991; Stechenberg, 1988).

The problem does not end with Lyme disease, however. Ticks carry all sorts of nasty bacteria, many of which can cause significant simultaneous difficulties that often get lumped in with Lyme disease. Babesiosis, Ehrlichiosis, Bartonella, and a host of other diseases can be carried and transmitted by ticks. As such, the co-infection rate of Lyme with other bacteria is quite high (Berghoff, 2012). These infectious diseases are often referred to collectively as tick-borne diseases (TBDs). Co-infections are particularly problematic because they may complicate diagnostic and treatment procedures.

How Common Is Lyme?

This question, like most having to do with Lyme, has no clear answer. Based on reports of laboratory testing, the Centers for Disease Control estimates that between 240,000 and 444,000 infections occurred in the United States in 2008. Based on medical claims to insurance companies between 2005 and 2010, the estimated number of people diagnosed with Lyme was between 296,000 and 376,000 per year. This represents approximately a tenfold increase of previous CDC estimates of infection rates. By any measure, this qualifies Lyme as a major public health concern (CDC, 2015).

The disease is not specific to the United States, however. Infection rates from various sources indicate the presence of TBDs in over 80 countries (Companion Vector Borne Diseases, 2013; Lyme Disease Association, 2013). According to the World Health Organization and the European Centre for Disease Control, the number of Lyme cases has been increasing steadily across Europe, with approximately 360,000 cases reported in the last two decades (WHO, ECDC, 2014).

This seems straightforward enough, but assessing the number of people infected with Lyme is complicated by the controversy over the guidelines that should be used for diagnosis. Many physicians reject the CDC diagnostic guidelines on the grounds that they are too stringent, thus underestimating the total number of actual cases. Additionally, there is controversy regarding the accuracy of the routine blood work to determine a diagnosis of Lyme disease, further clouding the diagnostic process and the calculations of Lyme's actual prevalence (Columbia University Medical Center, 2014). If any of these factors are at all relevant, the number of people infected with Lyme could be considerably higher than the CDC or WHO/ECDC statistics suggest.

What is clear is that the incidence of Lyme has increased considerably over the years. This is due to multiple factors. As additional lands become developed and people live and are active in more rural areas surrounded by woods and the creatures that live in them, the risk of exposure and infection increases. Lyme has been receiving considerable attention in the media of late for all of these reasons and others, fueling greater emphasis and attention on the disease. In short, Lyme disease is the fastest-growing infectious disease in the country, and many physicians and public health officials consider it to be nothing short of an epidemic (Horowitz, 2013).

Symptom Presentation

Once the Lyme bacteria enter the bloodstream and infiltrate cells of the various bodily systems, symptoms will begin to appear. Often infection is accompanied by a rash at the site of the tick bite called the erythema migrans (EM) or "bull's eye" rash, so named because it can look like a red bull's eye on the skin. The EM rash is used as criteria for a Lyme diagnosis, but it's not always present or it can be located in an undetectable area, such as under hair. While there are blood tests to determine the presence of Lyme, many physicians estimate that these routine blood tests can miss 35–50 percent of positive cases (Horowitz, 2013). The controversy regarding the accuracy of these tests means that a Lyme diagnosis is often made clinically, based predominantly on symptom presentation. Conversely, many physicians de-emphasize the clinical presentation and rely more heavily on the lab test results. This split in diagnostic criteria further adds to the confusion regarding the incidence of Lyme.

As you saw in Diane's case, the symptoms can be multi-systemic, quite varied in their presentation, and can be easily mistaken for a host of other problems. Symptoms of Lyme can include extreme fatigue, joint swelling/stiffness/pain, persistent headaches, sleep disturbance, mood disturbance (depression, mania), poor attention and/or concentration, cognitive impairment (difficulty thinking), sexual dysfunction, urinary symptoms, gastrointestinal problems, visual disturbances, irritability (sometimes leading to outbursts of rage), skin rashes, numbness or tingling sensations, Bell's palsy (facial drooping), anxiety or panic attacks, neurological impairment, swollen glands, fever, sore throat, unexplained back pain, muscle weakness, forgetfulness, speech errors or word-finding problems, psychosis, and light or sound sensitivity (Horowitz, 2013). Most people experience some cluster of these symptoms. As you can see, the potential disability caused by this illness is staggering.

Lyme Disease and Psychiatric Symptoms

The psychiatric implications of Lyme disease are poorly understood and not extensively researched. It is without question that Lyme disease can infiltrate and affect the body's nervous system, both central (brain and spinal cord) and peripheral (all other nerves in the body), meaning that Lyme can affect any of the body's voluntary or involuntary functions. The impacts of Lyme on various areas of functioning in the nervous system are well documented. There are extensive case examples of neuroborreliosis, the technical name for a Lyme infection of the nervous system, that illustrate the devastating impact of this condition.

What's less understood are the relationships among Lyme disease, depression, anxiety, mood swings, rage, and psychosis (Bransfield, 2012; Fallon et al, 1993; Fallon et al, 1995). This is an important topic that is worth some exploration because there's a powerful difference between being depressed or anxious because *you have a disease* versus being depressed or anxious *as a result of the disease*. There are many case examples to support the existence of mental illnesses as a symptom of Lyme rather than a consequence of it. However, differentiating between these possible causes of psychiatric symptoms can be very difficult, if not impossible. This is particularly important for mental and behavioral health professionals who work in tick-endemic areas and may encounter symptom presentations that look like psychiatric conditions but may actually be medically driven by the Lyme (or other TBDs) bacteria in the nervous system. It is also important if you're suffering from the illness to know and understand the difference to the best of your ability so you can make the best possible decisions regarding your care.

Pay Attention to Your Mental Health

If you're having psychiatric symptoms, there are important things to look for to help determine if Lyme might be a factor. Do you have an unusual symptom presentation? Are your symptoms new? Was there a sudden onset? Do you remain unresponsive to traditional treatment? For example, if you suddenly become depressed with no history of these problems, any triggering events, or changes in your life that would explain your shift in mood, it may be worth investigating Lyme as a potential factor, especially if you live in a tick-endemic area, recall a tick bite, or have any other symptoms consistent with Lyme.

Lyme-driven anxiety tends to last for longer periods of time compared to regular anxiety. For example, the typical panic attack generally lasts for 10–15 minutes with some aftereffects from the adrenaline rush being present for another hour or so. But Lyme-driven panic or intense anxiety can last for hours or days and typically comes in waves. Also, it's often not accompanied by dysfunctional or distorted thought processes as is usually the case with psychologically driven anxiety. Likewise, Lyme-driven symptoms (in my experience) tend to be less responsive to tried and true therapeutic interventions like cognitive behavioral or interpersonal therapy techniques. Therapists often become frustrated and puzzled by these cases, further enhancing your feelings of isolation and helplessness.

Don't get me wrong. I am NOT suggesting that all mental illness or psychiatric symptoms are Lyme driven. Mental illnesses have multifaceted causes that science does not fully understand. You can certainly become depressed and/or anxious for a whole host of reasons, not the least of which being that your life has been turned upside down by an illness. But Lyme may be a bit different in this regard because the bacteria can actually disrupt functioning in the nervous system and cause the symptoms itself. Looking for sudden onset, unusual presentations, simultaneous presentation of other Lyme symptoms, and unresponsiveness to treatment can be extraordinarily helpful and important in guiding diagnostic and treatment decision-making processes.

Taking all of this into account, it's critically important that you find a clinician who will do a thorough and detailed history and remain open to other possible causes of your presenting problem while also not automatically assuming that the symptoms are Lyme driven. This can be an incredibly difficult balance to strike, and this dynamic severely complicates the Lyme controversy. Obviously, there's nothing to prevent people with pre-existing mental illness from getting Lyme disease, but this does not mean that all cases of chronic Lyme are really psychiatric illnesses.

Conversely, not all psychiatric or medical conditions are caused by undiagnosed Lyme disease, but this almost certainly occurs as well. It's telling the difference that can be so difficult.

What Can You Do for Your Health?

From your perspective, it is paramount to remain open to receiving mental health services. The notion of doing this might not be very appealing to you. You know you're medically ill but might be getting the message from others that "it's all in your head," so the idea of seeing a psychologist or a psychiatrist seems like giving up and confirming the perception that you're "crazy."

However, avoiding engaging with mental health services because of this perspective can have unfortunate consequences. Knowledgeable or open-minded mental health professionals can often be powerful allies in helping you advocate for your health and can play a critical role in determining the cause of your symptoms as well as helping you decide the appropriate course of treatment. To illustrate the importance and complexities of differentiating the nature of psychiatric symptoms, we can look at the case example for Eddie, who came to me well before I became knowledgeable about Lyme disease.

Lyme-Driven Psychiatric Symptoms Case Example: Eddie

Eddie was a 33-year-old man who originally came to me for treatment several years prior to his Lyme diagnosis. He was having difficulty with anxiety and panic associated with a recently ended traumatic relationship. He was also quite perfectionistic and had obsessive compulsive personality tendencies, but that did not seem to be affecting his current functioning. His anxiety and panic remitted nicely with a course of exposure therapy, so treatment was terminated. A year or so later he returned to treatment for help with occupational difficulties and family issues. In the midst of this treatment, he was bitten by a tick and received a standard three-dose antibiotic treatment.

As we worked together in therapy, his condition worsened considerably. He began having severe mood swings, intense anxiety, and episodes of extreme rage that led to him running over a mailbox with his car and kicking a car in a store parking lot that resulted in legal ramifications. He also had significant fatigue, soreness in his joints, and light and noise sensitivity. He became intensely suicidal and was psychiatrically hospitalized several times.

Because of the rapid and severe worsening of his symptoms and functioning in conjunction with a recent tick bite, we eventually explored the possibility of his having contracted Lyme disease. He tested negative on the standard Lyme tests, but more sensitive testing indicated several positive bands for Lyme and other TBDs. He saw a Lyme specialist and began intensive antibiotic treatments, which eventually helped to relieve his symptoms.

Eddie's Diagnosis

Eddie's case is a complicated one. He had pre-existing mental health issues. But the intense and rapid change in his symptoms with no apparent cause as well as his unresponsiveness to psychotherapy and psychiatric medications were indications that something else may have been going on. Couple this with other Lyme symptoms and a known tick bite, and it made sense to start thinking that Lyme was a possible cause for his problems even though he had received the recommended antibiotic treatment at the time of the tick bite. It would have been very easy for any mental health professional to assume he was simply developing bipolar disorder and have him treated as such. Eddie's case illustrates the importance of remaining open to multiple causes of symptoms and for fast, accurate testing and appropriate treatment.

Treating Lyme Symptoms

As with most bacterial infections, the treatment of choice for Lyme disease is a course of appropriate antibiotics. Most would agree that if the disease is caught early and adequately treated, Lyme presents much fewer difficulties and can be relatively well controlled if not altogether cured. However, as Diane and Eddie's cases show us, if the symptoms are not recognized and treated quickly, the bacteria may spread and take a deeper hold in the body, making it more complex and difficult to treat. This is where much of the controversy surrounding Lyme exists. Many physicians believe that if the illness is not quickly and properly diagnosed and treated then treatment becomes considerably more difficult. Others disagree. If medicine can't agree on the diagnostic criteria, testing, and treatment procedures, then this increases the likelihood of missed or inaccurate diagnoses, potentially causing greater impairment, suffering, and disability.

Understanding the genesis of this controversy and its consequences is critically important to the management of this illness. The opposing positions of two medical societies perfectly illustrate the difficulties associated with diagnosing and treating Lyme disease. I strongly encourage anyone who has Lyme in their lives—patients, family members, caregivers, or health professionals—to further explore these issues and come to your own conclusions. However, I will offer a brief explanation of the controversy.

IDSA and ILADS

The Infectious Disease Society of America (IDSA) and the International Lyme and Associated Diseases Society (ILADS) are the two major groups of physicians on the front lines of the Lyme controversy. For the purposes of full disclosure, I mention here that I am a member of ILADS, but as I stated earlier, the purpose of this chapter is not to convince anyone of any particular point of view. It's simply to illustrate the existence of a very serious problem by informing you about the history of this controversy and how it may affect your approach (or your doctor's approach) to your illness.

The IDSA is the governing body of infectious disease doctors in the United States. Effectively, this means they are charged with developing treatment guidelines for the various infectious diseases based on the latest and best scientific evidence available. Once those guidelines are developed and disseminated, they become the de facto reference for the standard of treatment for all medical professionals when encountering that disease. In other words, when the IDSA developed and published *The Clinical Assessment, Treatment, and Prevention of Lyme Disease, Human Granulocytic Anaplasmosis, and Babesiosis: Clinical Practice Guidelines* (Wormser et al, 2006), this document became the standard for doctors across the country on how to diagnose and treat Lyme disease.

Not everyone agreed on the decisions made by the IDSA panel, including a group of physicians (who eventually formed ILADS) and the Connecticut Attorney General at the time, Richard Blumenthal. Because several members of the IDSA panel had affiliations with insurance companies, their conflicts of interest were called into question. Additionally, many physicians believed a strong portion of the scientific literature available at the time was not adequately considered by the panel, specifically in regard to the potential chronicity of the illness. The fervor around this eventually became so intense that Mr. Blumenthal initiated an anti-trust investigation of the IDSA panel. This investigation was eventually dropped based on mutual agreement that the guidelines be re-evaluated by a separate panel of specialists (Infectious Disease News, 2008).

In the meantime, the voice and membership of ILADS has grown considerably, so much so that ILADS has published its own set of guidelines for the treatment of Lyme disease. You don't have to be a physician to see the differences between the

IDSA and ILADS recommendations regarding the diagnosis and treatment of Lyme. For example, the IDSA guidelines suggest that anyone who has symptoms for longer than 6 weeks who has never been treated with antibiotics is unlikely to have Lyme disease if the blood test is negative, that most cases of Lyme disease are successfully treated with a few weeks of antibiotics, and that using antibiotics for a very long time (months or years) does not offer superior results (Wormser et al, 2006). The 2006 guidelines are, however, currently being updated.

Regarding the very same issues, the ILADS "Quick Facts About Lyme" page states, "The common ELISA test you receive at your doctor's office misses 35% of culture proven Lyme disease. Some studies indicate up to 50% of the patients tested for Lyme disease receive false negative results." Regarding the potential chronicity of the disease, ILADS says that "short treatment courses have resulted in upwards of a 40% relapse rate, especially if treatment is delayed. There has never been a study demonstrating that 30 days of antibiotic treatment cures chronic Lyme disease. However, there is much documentation demonstrating that short courses of antibiotic treatment fail to eradicate the Lyme spirochete" (ILADS). A more in-depth analysis of the ILADS treatment guidelines (Cameron, Johnson, and Maloney, 2014) shows stark differences in approaches to diagnosing and treating Lyme and other TBDs between the two medical organizations.

Conflict in Practice

Confusing, isn't it? The impact of these differences goes far beyond intellectual discourse. As mentioned earlier, the IDSA issues the guidelines for Lyme diagnosis and treatment. As such, most physicians approach the diagnosis and treatment of Lyme disease from the IDSA perspective, and understandably so. If I were a physician, to whom else would I turn for guidance in treating an infectious disease other than the governing body of the profession? Additionally, if I learned of a physician who was treating a patient outside those guidelines, in fact, in direct contradiction to those guidelines, it would be my professional responsibility to report that physician to my state's medical licensing board for further investigation. This is exactly what has happened to many physicians who treat Lyme under the ILADS guidelines.

In essence, ILADS physicians practice outside the IDSA-established guidelines of the profession in their treatment of Lyme because they fundamentally believe the guidelines to be flawed. However, they practice at great risk from other often well-intentioned physicians who are concerned about the excessive use of antibiotics and report doctors using the ILADS treatment protocol, making them subject to expensive and burdensome medical licensing board investigations. In short, physicians aligned with the ILADS perspective on Lyme practice at very high risk of professional and legal repercussions (this varies depending on state regulations where the physician practices, but you get the idea). The consequences of this are profound. There are far fewer physicians willing to practice under ILADS guidelines due to the risk. Because their services are often not reimbursed by insurance companies, seeing these physicians often becomes an out-of-pocket expense for patients seeking treatment. Additionally, if you tried to make a few phone calls to get an appointment with an ILADS physician, you know that the waiting lists are extremely long, sometimes 6–18 months. Thus, should one choose to seek this kind of treatment, it can be very difficult to access.

The impact of this for people suffering from Lyme is nothing short of staggering. What you have are two medical societies arguing vehemently over the most basic facts regarding an illness, legions of physicians who are following guidelines that may or may not be accurate, and patients who are extremely sick, disabled, and often dismissed as having symptoms that are "all in their heads." There are countless examples of people who were not adequately treated by mainstream medicine but who recovered to normal functioning once receiving treatment from a physician with an ILADS perspective on the illness. Conversely, many who get ILADS-based treatment do not recover well and continue to suffer. Ultimately, anecdotal evidence will not resolve any of these issues, but the science surrounding these issues has been painstakingly slowed by the politics.

ACT and the Lyme Trap

Practically speaking, people with Lyme have a tough road to navigate to figure out what kind of medical treatment they want to receive and how to access it. These are decisions that each and every person has to make for themselves. You would like to simply trust the medical community to let you know what the best course of action is. However, as you can see, for some reason that simply hasn't happened for Lyme disease, at least not yet.

I can assure you, trying to figure all of this out when you're healthy and well is difficult enough. A brief perusal of academic databases for scientifically based information quickly reveals a sharp division along the lines outlined above. The language used in much of the writing about this topic is frequently inflammatory and it makes it excruciatingly difficult to figure out what exactly is going on. Most of us are not trained scientists or medical professionals, so wading through the different studies and approaches is a daunting task under the best of circumstances, let alone when you're extremely ill and compromised.

This illustrates the first "logistical" aspect of the Lyme Trap—figuring out what to do and then how to do it in regard to getting treatment for your illness. There are conflicting messages and disagreements from the medical community about every major aspect of Lyme disease, not the least of which are guidelines for diagnosis and treatment. If you want to feel trapped, try figuring out what to do about your medical condition when the medical community itself cannot agree on what you should do. It can be very difficult to effect any real control over your situation.

As I mentioned before, there have been many books written about this aspect of Lyme disease, but that's not what this book is about. I covered this material only to make you aware of its existence. I can't provide definitive answers about this for you. Frankly, I don't have a medical degree or the technical background to answer those questions, so I'll leave that to others to resolve. I can only make observations about what I see Lyme patients experiencing and the scientific discourse surrounding the issues. Fortunately, however, there are aspects of the Lyme Trap over which you do have control.

Taking Control Where You Can: ACT in Action

This book is focused on helping you deal with the second aspect of the Lyme Trap, which is far more internal and something over which you actually do have some influence. As we've seen, Lyme can be a devastating illness that can stop you in your tracks and turn your life upside down. It can keep your body and mind from working properly in a variety of ways.

Because of your illness, you may find yourself putting everything about your life on hold until you're feeling well again. This is a natural and understandable reaction. You feel exhausted, you can't think clearly, and you're in pain. Of course you have to wait until you're feeling better to do the things that you like or that need to be done. Unfortunately, the nature of the disease may leave you with a longer wait than you would prefer until you're feeling better, and with some chronic diseases, you may never feel 100 percent like yourself again. That's a terrifying thought, but this book is designed to help you with exactly that problem.

The internal aspect of the Lyme Trap is falling victim to putting your life on hold until you're over your illness, whether it be Lyme or some other chronic medical condition. It's natural for anyone, for you, to think about living your life only when you are well again. But what if you can live your life in a better way than you are living it right now even though you're still sick? This is the essence and purpose of this book, to learn how to live in the best way possible despite the fact that you may be feeling your worst. You may have an illness that has wreaked havoc on your life, but you can take some of that life back.

Transform Your Suffering, No Matter the Cause

The good news is that in order to benefit from this book, you don't have to answer the question of whether or not you have Lyme disease—or Multiple Sclerosis, or Chronic Fatigue Syndrome, or Fibromyalgia, or some other illness, including medical problems that are supposedly "all in your head." The bottom line is that you're suffering, and *that* is what this book is designed to help you with, regardless of where that suffering comes from. As I stated earlier, this book is not about curing you of your illness. It's about living your life to its fullest possible potential while you get well even though you may not be thinking or feeling like you can. It's not just about escaping the Lyme Trap; it's about not being trapped at all.

Needless to say, this is a tall order to fill and is much easier said than done, but I believe that through mindfulness and ACT tools you can live a better life while your life gets better. Fundamentally, ACT is an approach designed to help you deal with suffering, including distress caused by acute, chronic, and devastating illnesses. While this book is written specifically for people with Lyme disease, your ability to benefit from what's presented in the pages that follow has absolutely nothing to do with whether or not your doctor has diagnosed you with Lyme or thinks you're a hypochondriac. In other words, the approaches in this book should be effective for you regardless of the medical controversy surrounding Lyme in general or your case specifically. Ultimately, you are in control of how you deal with your pain and suffering, no matter its origins or what others may think might be causing it.

I hope you're willing to explore the possibility that your life, even with an illness, can be more than what it is now. You may not be quite sure how that can happen, but I've seen it work in my own practice and I've seen the empirical data about the overall effectiveness of ACT. It's possible to live vitally and meaningfully regardless of how we might feel or why we might feel that way.

Chapter 2

Acceptance and Commitment Therapy

Do you want to know who you are? Don't ask. Act! Action will delineate and define you.
Thomas Jefferson

ACT: What's It All About?

ACT, at its core, is about dealing with human suffering. More specifically, it's about creating a different relationship with whatever pain and difficulty you have in your life, a relationship that allows you to move forward and live to the best of your ability rather than continuously struggle with avoiding or vanquishing pain. As human beings, we're naturally inclined to avoid and escape physical and emotional discomfort. It makes perfect sense. It's part of our survival instinct and has kept us alive for thousands of years. But sometimes that survival mechanism causes more problems than it prevents. When we become so focused on avoiding pain, we end up not actually living our lives at all but expending all of our energy on trying to create a pain-free life. This simply isn't realistic or possible.

A fundamental principle of ACT is that we can coexist with pain. The greatest difficulties in our lives come from our attempts to avoid pain through maladaptive and dysfunctional behavior (Hayes et al, 2012). Our culture has become brainwashed by the idea that we're supposed to be happy all of the time and that if we aren't then something's wrong with us that requires some sort of intervention—be it medication, therapy, or distraction. The classic example of this is the alcoholic who chooses to drink in an attempt to avoid whatever emotional pain he may be experiencing. At some point, simply choosing to experience that pain would be much less destructive and difficult than the havoc, chaos, and damage wrought by excessive drinking and avoidance.

You don't have to be an alcoholic or drug abuser to be excessively avoidant. We avoid pain in a variety of ways. We watch too much TV instead of exercising. We get involved in destructive relationships because we don't want to face being alone. We engage excessively with technology to avoid the discomfort of real human contact. We keep others at a distance with our anger or irritability. We don't go for the job promotion because we don't want to deal with the possible embarrassment of not getting it. While this all might help us to lead a "safe" life and create the illusion of being pain free, the reality is that we're leading lives that lack the richness, vitality, and meaning we truly desire.

Emotions, by their very nature, are transient. They come and they go, so if we make decisions in our lives based solely on emotional consequences then our decisions are constantly changing and directionless. We never really get where we want to go, and we end up running around in circles. The ultimate result of all of this is that while we may have the illusion of feeling safe, we are not actually pain free.

I spend a lot of time in my private practice helping people realize that the real reason they have to see me, the real reason they're having so many problems in their lives, is that they're spending too much of their time and energy avoiding pain, and this is what actually causes their suffering. As we will see, pain and suffering are not the same thing. Pain is unavoidable in life. It's part of the human experience. But suffering is a result of how we deal with pain. The alcoholic *suffers* because he drinks to avoid his pain. If he chose simply to experience his pain, to coexist with it, to create a less threatening relationship with it rather than avoid it through alcohol use, then he wouldn't be suffering. In pain? Yes. But suffering? No.

ACT is about letting go of the idea that we can live pain-free lives. If we accept that we will experience pain, we can let go of our suffering. This is a counterintuitive but powerful approach to life that requires a willingness to do things differently and try something that might not immediately feel comfortable but will eventually lead to a better and more functional life. If ACT is about suffering, then people who are trying to live with Lyme or any chronic illness need ACT because it's designed exactly for situations over which we have little or no control.

The History of ACT

A full account of the history of ACT and its theoretical underpinnings is beyond the scope of this book and, frankly, more than most people would want to read. The good news is that it doesn't matter much if you don't understand the science behind it. All that matters is that you know there *is* science behind it. ACT is not a fly-by-night fad treatment that will come and go. I don't think you'll ever be seeing any infomercials about it. That said, it's worth understanding a bit about where it comes from and its place in the science of psychology.

In the early days of psychology, the dominant theoretical approach to treating psychological problems was Psychoanalysis, created by Sigmund Freud (Mitchell and Black, 1996). Psychoanalysis focuses almost entirely on unconscious processes and conflicts, the idea being that if there are unresolved issues lurking around your unconscious mind, those conflicts will manifest themselves by way of a psychological disorder, be it depression, anxiety, or another form of pathology (Freud, 1995). There is no denying Freud's place in the history of the field, but his theories have been roundly criticized for their lack of scientific evidence (Szasz and Kraus, 1990).

Largely as a reaction to Freud's theories, a group of behavioral scientists started studying observable behavior rather than unconscious processes. By the middle of the twentieth century, largely due to the work of iconic psychologist B. F. Skinner, the dominant psychological theory of the time was Behaviorism, which focused on the study of observable behavior. To facilitate change, these scientists targeted the consequences of behavior (Skinner, 1976). This is where the concepts of reinforcement and punishment were born in order to increase or decrease the frequency of a certain behavior (Skinner, 1965).

Eventually, the idea of introducing conscious thought as a determining factor in human behavior made its way into Behaviorism, and thus Cognitive Behavioral Therapy (CBT) was born (Beck and Beck, 2011). CBT is often referred to as the "second wave" of behavioral therapy and has become the dominant form of treatment for a variety of psychological disorders. It's exceptionally effective and has massive amounts of scientific evidence to support its therapeutic value. CBT focuses on changing the nature of one's thoughts from predominantly negative and dysfunctional to more neutral, positive, or rational. When this is accomplished then changes in emotions and/or behavior follow, thus alleviating suffering on the part of the patient (Beck and Beck, 2011).

I was trained in CBT my entire career and was a diehard disciple of the model. I witnessed firsthand its effectiveness in treating a variety of psychological difficulties. However, for all of the success I had using CBT, I would often find myself "hitting a wall" in treatment, particularly when I was helping people who weren't necessarily having dysfunctional thoughts but had exceptionally difficult life problems like chronic illness. My use of the CBT model felt lacking in these kinds of situations. These are the types of situations in which I believe ACT excels.

The advent of ACT, which has been over 30 years in the making, is considered part of the "third wave" of behavioral therapies (Hayes et al, 2012). It's grounded in an extremely well researched model called Relational Frame Theory, which focuses on how our minds form relations and use symbols and language to make connections in our mental processes (Hayes, Barnes-Holmes, and Roche, 2001). This is a remarkably adaptive human skill, but can also get us stuck in some negative feedback loops that underlie a lot of psychopathology.

The ACT model itself has become more and more mainstream in the last 10 to 15 years. It is not without its criticisms, but the founders of the model and those who practice it tend to be scientifically minded, open to criticism, and have a genuine desire to move ACT in whatever direction the science and the data take it. There have been over 100 randomized clinical trials (the gold standard of scientific investigation) testing the effectiveness of the model.

ACT is part of a larger movement of psychotherapeutic approaches called Contextual Behaviorism or Contextual Behavioral Science (Hayes et al, 2013). Specifically, ACT is a model that adheres to Functional Contextualism. To keep this very simple, Functional Contextualism is all about doing what works (functional), when and where it works (context). Functional Contextual approaches refuse to judge or categorize behavior outside the context in which the behavior occurs and without understanding the function of the behavior (Biglan and Hayes, 1996).

For example, ACT is not *always* against experiential avoidance. If you step off the curb and a car is speeding towards you, it's perfectly acceptable to avoid the experience of getting hit by that car. Similarly, ACT would never advocate that anyone who is the victim of domestic abuse learn to "accept" the abuse. Behavior occurs in the context of larger value systems and needs to be evaluated within these contexts. As an ACT practitioner, I would never discourage a client from seeking appropriate medical care and to simply "accept" their illness *unless it was part of their articulated value system*. I don't determine those contexts or values; I only help clients discover them for themselves.

Ultimately, ACT will ask you to do things that seem different but will have powerful results. In order to accomplish forming this new relationship with your pain and discomfort, you need to increase your psychological flexibility. This is a core, fundamental goal of ACT.

Psychological Flexibility

ACT's approach to human suffering is to increase psychological flexibility, which is the ability to contact the present moment more fully as a conscious human being and to change or persist in behavior when doing so serves valued ends (Hayes et al, 2012). So, what does this mean exactly? *Contact with the present moment* means that you're aware of and in touch with whatever experiences you're having, especially emotionally, at each moment in time. Psychological inflexibility is the opposite of this and consists of engaging in avoidance to escape the present moment because the present moment might be painful or undesirable. A psychologically flexible person is able to stay in contact with the present even if that present is uncomfortable, difficult, or painful.

Changing or persisting in behavior to serve valued ends means that we make decisions about what we do or don't do based NOT on attempts to avoid pain or discomfort but on what will move us towards what we truly value and matters most to us. Psychological flexibility simply allows us to feel what we feel when we feel it and do what we need to do in order to move towards our values *regardless of our emotional or physical experiences.*

Psychological flexibility requires us to be open, centered, and engaged. ACT has six core processes to facilitate movement in this direction. Each of these six core processes is described in great detail in the following chapters of this book, but I will briefly cover them here to give you a picture of the model as a whole.

The Six Core Processes to Being Open, Centered, and Engaged:

1. Defusion > Open
2. Acceptance > Open

3. Self-As-Context > Centered
4. Contact with the Present Moment > Centered
5. Values > Engaged
6. Committed Action > Engaged

In following chapters, I'll give you specific exercises to practice these skills and increase your psychological flexibility.

Being Open

Being open is about freeing yourself from the struggle to avoid, extinguish, enhance, or otherwise control your emotions. It involves giving yourself over to the moment-to-moment experience of your thoughts and feelings, recognizing that this is simply part of being human, that all thoughts and emotions are, by their very nature, transient. As such, making decisions about what you do with your life based on these transient states or, worse yet, spending all of your time trying to control something that's ever-changing, is actually what leads to suffering. Being open involves the core processes of Defusion and Acceptance.

Defusion

As human beings, we are *always* thinking. As you read these words, there's a verbal script running through your head making comments about what you're reading, thinking about other things you need to do, worrying about your illness, etc. ACT refers to this process as actions of the "mind." We have the amazing ability to think about what we are thinking about, which is adaptive and sets us apart from all other species. Unfortunately, we also have the tendency to automatically believe everything we think and become "fused" with that thought process.

In other words, we tend to let our thoughts dominate and dictate the experience of our lives, which can lead to dysfunction. Defusion is about observing our own thought processes, recognizing that our thoughts are just that—thoughts—and that we have the ability to make decisions about how we engage with our thoughts. Defusion does NOT encourage attempts to control our thought processes because this is futile, drains our energy, and engages us in an unnecessary struggle, taking us away from values-driven action.

Acceptance

Acceptance is probably the most misunderstood core process of ACT—I am going to ask that you be patient with it. Chapter 4 will provide much more insight into the ACT version of acceptance, which is different from what most people think of when they hear the word "acceptance." People confuse it with giving up or tolerating a difficult experience. That belief leads to a resistance to this process in general and especially for people with chronic illness. In ACT, acceptance is the alternative to experiential avoidance and involves being open to experiencing the private events of your life, including your illness. This is NOT to say that acceptance discourages you from getting well. On the contrary, the whole idea of acceptance is to *live well while you're getting well*, which is the entire point of this book.

For example, acceptance asks you to be open to feeling whatever you're feeling—anxiety, depression, pain, despair—fully and without defense or struggle. It is the antithesis of avoidance. It allows us to release our futile attempts at controlling our emotions and put that energy into other more values-based activities whether they be seeking treatment, connecting with a loved one, engaging in a leisure activity, or simply resting. Acceptance in ACT is not an end in itself or a goal to be achieved. It's a process designed to foster and increase values-based actions.

Being Centered

The second domain of ACT focuses on being centered with your experience of the moment. The circumstances of our lives tend to pull us into the past or the future, feeding uncomfortable emotions like anxiety, regret, fear, and despair. By remaining centered on our experience of the moment, we remove much of the fuel of these energy-draining emotions. Being centered involves the core ACT processes of Self-As-Context and Contact with the Present Moment.

Self-As-Context

People suffering from chronic Lyme have a tendency to over-identify with their illness. Because the disease can be so debilitating, Lyme becomes your life and you lament the loss of what was probably an active, vibrant existence. Lyme overwhelms your sense of self. Rather than having a life in which you experience Lyme disease, Lyme disease becomes the life you experience. This is often complicated by excessive focus on "who you were" and "hope to be once again," losing or rejecting your actual self in the process.

In other words, you are defining yourself in terms of the *content* of your life rather than the *context* of your life. This "self-as-content" approach leads to a poor foundation and allows for too much definition of the self by the events of your life. Self-as-context, on the other hand, allows you to maintain your sense of self. You are who you are in this moment in time—your experience is only the context in which you experience yourself. The content of your life doesn't define you—it's merely the environment in which your life is happening. Through an emphasis on self-as-context rather than self-as-content, you can rediscover who you are in the context of having an illness rather than defining yourself by it.

Contact with the Present Moment

While ACT recognizes that at times we must plan for the future and remember the past, it's beneficial for the majority of our life experience to be dominated by our connection with the present moment because it's the only aspect of our lives over which we can exert any control. ACT promotes open, non-judgmental contact with the present experience of your life no matter how difficult, uncomfortable, painful, joyous, exhilarating, or devastating that feeling may be. By remaining present, you only experience the emotions of the moment and abdicate any attempt to control your emotions of the past or the future. Being present hones and focuses your attention. Being in this space allows you to be more flexible and to make decisions that will move the direction of your life towards what you value.

The process of mindfulness is central to being present. Mindfulness is a centuries-old practice that has taken on different meanings in different contexts. In ACT, mindfulness is simply giving your full attention to your experience of the present moment. It is a vitally important process in the ACT model.

Being Engaged

ACT is an approach to life that is rooted in behavior. It's about *doing*. There is only so much discussion, thinking, deliberating, and understanding that can happen. If real change is going to happen in any context, that change will have to happen as a result of engaging in your life to the best of your ability. Waiting until problems pass—waiting until you are no longer sick to live your life—will lead to a life unfulfilled, more pain, and more suffering. ACT encourages you to engage with your life no matter the circumstances to the best of your ability at any given point in time, recognizing that engagement may lead to pain or uncomfortable circumstances. But if that pain is in service of moving you forward, then this is an acceptable—maybe even necessary—pain. Turning away from it only delays your life. The two core processes of psychological flexibility that facilitate being engaged are Values and Committed Action.

Values

I spend a lot of time with clients helping them understand that avoiding pain and discomfort in their lives is often a futile and counterproductive exercise—that making decisions based on avoiding or chasing an emotional experience will lead to living your life in circles, doing the same things over and over again. The question inevitably arises, "If I don't make decisions based on what I think or what I feel, then how do I decide what to do?" I love this question because it's my cue to help my clients discover their values and lead a life guided by the things that are truly important to them. It usually represents a real "a-ha" moment in treatment.

Values are the freely chosen, purposeful directions we take in our life. They serve as constant guideposts to the decisions we make about our behavior. At any given time, we are either engaged in behavior that is moving us towards what we value or behavior that is keeping us from it. Values are not goals to be attained, but rather criteria upon which to base our decisions.

For example, being a father is a goal. It's an attainable thing, but being a *good* father is a value. I am never done being a good father (hopefully). I don't suddenly reach "good father" status and my job is over. For the rest of my life, my value of being a good father is a factor in every decision I make. Sometimes being a good parent hurts. I don't enjoy punishing my kids, but I have to endure that discomfort in order for my kids to learn how to behave properly and function as productive and contributing members of society. If I avoided the discomfort of punishing them by not doing so, what would happen to my children? What would the emotional consequence of that avoidance be for me? For them?

ACT is not a sadistic model that asks you to suck it up and endure pain, but it does ask you to accept that pain is a necessary part of leading a values-driven life. If that pain is in service of moving you towards a value—whatever that value may be—

then you're moving your life forward, engaging in whatever you can, and leading a richer, more vital existence. Discovering your values is an absolute necessity in ACT as those values become the guiding beacons in all of your decision-making processes.

Committed Action

As mentioned previously, ACT is grounded in Behaviorism. Ultimately it is about *doing*, and this is where committed action comes in. ACT advocates taking committed action towards your values at all times with full acknowledgment and acceptance of the fact that this action may expose you to difficult or uncomfortable emotions, feelings, or sensations. It also gives you the necessary tools to be psychologically flexible enough not to let pain or discomfort affect your decisions or your behavior in a way that moves you away from your values.

Inevitably, in the work I do with clients, we get to a point where they're frustrated—they're open, they're centered, but only partially engaged. This is the "just do it" phase of the process, and it's an absolute necessity for progress. For people with Lyme and chronic illness, it should be noted that often "just do it" involves resting, caring for yourself, and choosing NOT to do a particular thing because the resulting consequence may lead to a setback, cause more harm than good, or maybe just isn't possible in the moment. Sometimes acceptance of this process can be more difficult than anything.

The Hexaflex

Taken as a whole, each of these processes supports the others to improve psychological flexibility, allowing you to contact the present moment fully and make choices in the service of chosen values. The figure overleaf (Figure 2.1) is known as the "Hexaflex," a diagrammatic representation of the ACT model. While I understand this type of diagram can be intimidating or overwhelming at first, hang in there. For now, just take a look at it without any pressure to "get it" — we'll circle back to it later and "bring it home" after you have a better sense of the core processes.

As you can see, each core process is connected to and affected by the other. None of them occurs in isolation and all are in support of the core process of psychological flexibility. ACT is not linear. You don't learn defusion, then acceptance, then self-as-context and so forth. If you're engaged in acceptance, you're also engaged in values and committed action. Each process accounts for all of the other processes in the model at all times. It's a fluidly functioning way to engage with your life. We'll get into that much more in Chapter 9.

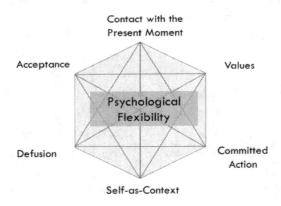

Figure 2.1: The Hexaflex Model of Psychological Flexibility
(reprinted with permission from Hayes et al, 2012)

Psychological Inflexibility

To look at it another way, psychological inflexibility is dominated by the opposite of the core ACT processes—fusion with your thoughts, experiential avoidance, dominance of a conceptualized past and feared future, attachment to the conceptualized self (or self-as-content), an absence of values, inactivity, avoidance, or impulsivity. This pattern of behavior will lead to a life that is rigid, seized, inflexible, and unfulfilled as seen in Figure 2.2. This model will work just as fluidly to prevent you from moving your life forward and keeping your life stuck.

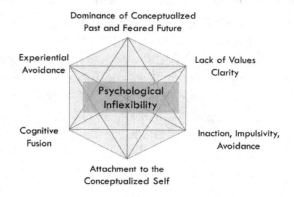

Figure 2.2: A Model of Psychological Inflexibility and Rigidity
(reprinted with permission from Hayes et al, 2012)

A Return to Mindfulness

A little bit ago, I mentioned mindfulness as a centrally important process in ACT, specifically in regard to contact with the present moment. Your ability to be mindful is the bedrock of successful implementation of ACT.

Mindfulness has been practiced for centuries by many cultures using a variety of different methods for countless purposes. It is perhaps most associated with Zen Buddhism and for good reason. Most people's basic understanding of mindfulness is drawn from their knowledge of Asian cultures and Buddhist teachings. It's this Eastern influence that's been incorporated into Western psychotherapy approaches led by Jon Kabat-Zinn, Ekhart Tolle, and many others (Williams and Kabat-Zinn, 2013). Mindfulness is often mistaken for religious practice. While it may be utilized in certain religious rituals or practices, ACT takes a secular approach to mindfulness.

Traditionally, Western psychotherapy has used relaxation

techniques to decrease anxiety and distress. This can be done with great success in many circumstances, but it can also be counterproductive. Some people will put pressure on themselves to be relaxed, and if they're not they think they're doing something wrong, which causes distress and anxiety, thus defeating the purpose. Relaxation techniques also inherently approach anxiety and distress as feelings to be reduced or eliminated. As we have seen, this is not what ACT seeks to do.

Think about it. If I'm anxious and undertake the task of engaging in a relaxation exercise, I am by the very nature of the process pitting relaxation against anxiety—a battle of my parasympathetic (the peaceful side) and sympathetic (stressful side) nervous systems. What we know about our nervous systems and our minds is that anytime we see something as a "battle," it tends to trigger our fight-or-flight response. This then sends us off to the races, triggering all of the physiological symptoms of stress and anxiety. This doesn't happen all of the time of course, and I've had great success using relaxation techniques with clients in a variety of situations, but I have found that it has limitations that mindfulness approaches address quite nicely.

Mindfulness involves being in contact with the present moment fully and without judgment while acknowledging and accepting any emotional experiences or physical sensations that are occurring in the moment (Hayes et al, 2012). Mindfulness sidesteps the whole battle between relaxation and distress by simply acknowledging the presence of whatever is present—to simply bear witness to the unfolding events of your life, free of judgment and without attempts to influence or change them (Hayes and Smith, 2005).

Mindfulness can be a struggle because it's quite opposite to the way we're used to living our lives. The good news is that mindfulness is not some magical talent that some people have and some people don't. It's a skill. With practice, anyone can become more mindful. *You* can become more mindful, which will allow you to engage in the core processes of ACT and bring about radical change to your life. Below is a very simple, very basic, and very short mindfulness exercise that will provide a foundation for the advanced work we will be doing later in the book.

I recommend that you read through the following exercise a few times first to get a sense of what you'll be doing. You could also record the exercise and listen to it while you're engaging in it. How you do it is less important than actually doing it, however. As with all of the exercises in this book, I encourage you to do them, not just read them. Remember, ACT is about *doing*, so don't undermine what you can get from it by avoidance!

Mindfulness Exercise: Mindful Senses

Find a relatively quiet, comfortable place where you won't be interrupted. Turn off the radio or TV and set your phone to silent so you won't be too distracted. It doesn't have to be absolutely silent. Just do the best you can. For this exercise, I invite you to sit comfortably on a chair or a couch with your feet flat on the floor and your hands in your lap or at your side. You can close your eyes or keep them fixed on a specific point on the floor or the wall.

Take a few nice, easy breaths, one after another. As you breathe in, focus on how the cool air feels in your nose and mouth, moving down your windpipe and into your lungs...and as you breathe out, focus on how the warm air feels leaving your body. Just keep breathing for a little bit, focusing on those sensations of your breath. Now turn your attention to the rest of your senses. Focus on how the cushion feels against your legs...your back, your arms...how your hands feel in your lap or at your sides...focus on any sounds you might be able to hear, the heater or air conditioner blowing in the room, traffic noise outside the window, or the house settling. Just turn your attention to any sounds you might hear. Welcome the experience of the sound and focus on how it feels...the sound moving into your ear. On your next in-breath, notice if there are any smells in the air, and just breathe them in...focus on the quality of the smell, is it bitter or sweet, pleasant or unpleasant? Do you taste anything as you breathe in? Just breathe it in and let it become part of you. Now pay attention to your total sensory experience, everything you feel, smell, hear, taste, just allow those sensations to be there and focus on them. If you drift off and your mind wanders, that's okay, just gently acknowledge it and bring your full focus and attention back to your sensory experience. Now, take a moment to return to the focus on your breath, the coolness on the in-breath, the warmth of the out-breath. Just focus on that for a bit...and open your eyes when you feel ready and comfortable.

This is a very basic mindfulness exercise, but it carries with it a powerful tool in that your sensory experience is almost always present-focused. However ungrounded in the present you may feel, if you want to get yourself there, focusing on your sensory experiences is a good way to do it. If you're in pain from your illness, it carries with it the added benefit of a little bit of acceptance work (more on this in Chapter 4). Starting to do this exercise with any degree of regularity will serve as a great foundation for being more mindful in more difficult and triggering circumstances. If you found yourself wandering, I promise you that everyone who does this exercise, or any other mindfulness exercise, finds themselves wandering also. It's important not to judge yourself or be harsh. Just gently acknowledge that you stepped outside the moment and bring yourself back to the exercise. Practicing the process of just "coming back to center" is an invaluable exercise that will serve you well.

Psychological Flexibility and Lyme

ACT encourages you to engage in your life, no matter how difficult or painful that life might be in the moment. Improving your psychological flexibility allows you to sidestep the issues of whether or not you have Lyme, what your doctor thinks, and what your diagnosis is or isn't. Instead, ACT brings focus to your unique internal experience. While answering all of these questions will ultimately be important, you don't have to sacrifice your values or put your life on hold until you get those answers. On the contrary, ACT encourages you to engage with your life to the fullest of your ability at *every* moment.

Now that you have a bit of background and foundation about what ACT is and how it can help you transcend your suffering, it's time to build your experience with the six core processes of ACT. While there's nothing that will be "easy" about becoming more psychologically flexible, if you fully engage, it will be transformative.

Chapter 3

Don't Believe Everything You Think

There is nothing either good or bad, but thinking makes it so.
William Shakespeare

The Importance of Defusion

Human beings are thinking creatures. We're always doing it—as we're talking to people, listening to people, writing, reading, running errands. Chances are, if we're conscious (and sometimes even not) that little voice constantly running in the back of our minds is active and vocal. There's nothing wrong with this. It's just part of being human. What we have to recognize is that this voice, even though it's ours, doesn't have dominion over our lives. As mentioned in the previous chapter, we have a strong tendency to become fused with that voice (what ACT refers to as our "mind") and accept whatever it's telling us without question or doubt. It is, after all, *your* voice representing *your* thoughts, so how wrong could it be? As it turns out, it can often be quite destructive.

Your Thinking Self

Looking at the content of your mind (your thinking self) is nothing new in psychology. It's a hallmark approach in CBT to call that voice out for being irrational and wrestle it back to a more rational place, which under a wide range of circumstances can be very helpful. But what happens if a thought isn't really irrational? You've been afflicted with a debilitating disease. There's nothing irrational or dysfunctional about that. Your illness is not the product of your thinking mind; it's the product of a real medical condition. Thinking differently about it isn't necessarily going to change the nature of your circumstances.

ACT takes a slightly different approach to dealing with our thinking selves by focusing more on the function of our thoughts rather than whether they're right or wrong, rational or irrational, healthy or unhealthy.

Whenever you're thinking, you're using language. When you use language, you're using symbols (words) to create relations among the various events, objects, and emotions of your life. You relate Lyme to the devastation it's brought to your life. Naturally, Lyme, your life, and devastation become "related frames" in your mind. Remember in Chapter 2 when I briefly mentioned Relational Frame Theory as the foundation of ACT? Well, this is it in action. When we form these relations through symbolic representations (language) in our minds, accurate or not, they have a tendency to stick. In some cases, these relations save our lives. The last time you ate a berry off that bush, you got really sick. That relational frame will keep you from eating a berry from that bush again, but should it keep you from eating all berries from any bush ever?

In ACT, there's a recognition that sometimes our relational frames get tangled up, especially when dealing with emotions. That entanglement, or fusion, keeps us locked in our thinking selves and prevents us from being able to observe our own thought process. As such, we end up behaving in accordance with those relational frames—we never eat any berries from any bushes at all—and this inhibits us from being able to do things that might be good or necessary for our health and well-being. Many berries are valuable sources of nutrition, but if you remain fused with the thought "all berries will make me sick," you end up depriving yourself of the benefits of good, healthy berries.

Naturally, we don't really worry much about what berries are tasty or poisonous these days, but in other areas this kind of fusion with our thinking selves leads to significant dysfunction and experiential avoidance in our lives. Take a moment to reflect on what your mind tells you about the fact that you're sick right now. Do you have thoughts about how much less of a person you are? How you can't live your life the way you want to because you're sick? How your spouse or partner might not love you as much since you've become ill? That you are a burden to the people you love in your life because you can't do the things you used to do? I want you to actually get a pen and paper and make a list of the common thoughts you have about your Lyme. Set it aside for a bit. We'll come back to it.

This kind of fusion with our thoughts tends to happen across six different domains (Harris, 2009). Each is explained briefly below, but you should pay close attention to which domain resonates with you the most, especially in the context of your illness.

- **Rules**: Rule-governed thinking is relatively easy to catch once you recognize the cues. Any statements you make to yourself that contain *should, must, ought*, or *if-then* language are red flags. *I should be healthier or feeling better. If I were feeling better or weren't sick, then I'd be a better mother. I ought to be stronger and better able to do things.* These kinds of rule-governed thought patterns are inflexible and lend themselves to suffering.
- **Reasons**: Any time you find yourself coming up with reasons, or essentially excuses, for not engaging in values-driven behavior, you're engaging in reason-governed thinking. *I'm not strong enough to take care of my family because I'm sick* might be an example of reason-governed thinking that could hold you back from making meaningful life changes.
- **Judgments**: Negative or positive judgments of others or yourself often lead to fused thinking, self-fulfilling prophecies, disappointments, and inflexibility in your thought processes. *I'm no good at this, I'll never get well, this disease will run my life forever, other people are healthy*

and happy are all examples of unhelpful judgments.
- **Past and Future**: Fusion with positive or negative thoughts regarding the past or future compromises your ability to be flexible. If you're stuck in your thoughts about your past "healthy" life and convinced of your future of being ill, this can paralyze your present.
- **Self**: Thoughts about yourself are essentially stories you make up based on interpretations of your past experiences. *I'm sick. I'm weak. I'm tough.* Whatever the story may be, it lends itself to inflexibility in the present moment when your situation may call for an approach that's different from your conceptualized self.

This is where defusion becomes an important skill in the ACT process. The goal in defusion is to gain some separation from these processes and the stories you tell yourself about who you are and what you're capable of in order to be more flexible in your behavior and your actions in the present moment. You do this by tapping into your ability to be observant of your own thoughts.

Your Observing Self

ACT increases your ability to observe your own thought processes, giving you some separation between your thinking self and your observing self. As magical and wonderful as it is that our minds are always working, it's even more powerful when we use it to *observe* that process and make decisions about it. Note, I am not saying you have the ability to *control* or *stop* your mind. That's an endless and futile game, because in order to stop thinking about something, you have to think about it. Go ahead and try it. Close your eyes and try NOT to think about your Lyme symptoms. What happened? Predictably, you ended up thinking about your disease, didn't you? That's what happens when you try not to think about something—you end up engaging with the very thing you're trying not to think of. Any time you're struggling with something, it's inherently present in your life and in your mind because you're holding it there. Moreover, while you're caught in that struggle, you're being pulled away from other things that really matter to you.

This begs the question, if you can't push your thoughts out of your head, control them, or make them go away, then what do you do with them? This is where the observing self and defusion play a vital role. Since we have the ability to observe our thought processes, we also have the ability to decide how much or how little we want to engage with those thoughts. While you may not be able to *control* your mind or your thoughts, you do have the ability to control *what you do* surrounding those thoughts, just like you can't control other people but you can control how you react to them. Again, the idea behind defusion is to create separation between your thinking self and observing self—*not to control your thoughts*. In other words, have whatever thoughts you're having, but observe the fact that you are having them and carry them with you lightly while you forge ahead and do what really matters to you (Wilson and DuFrene, 2010).

What does this mean exactly? Well, let's say you have a disturbing thought about your illness. Go ahead and pick one from that list you made a little bit ago. For the purposes of the exercise, I'll use the thought about being a burden to your loved ones. This is a difficult and disturbing thought to have. No one wants to be a burden to the people they love, so the natural inclination is to try and push this thought away or get rid of it somehow. You may try to distract yourself or seek reassurance from your family with comments like *I'm sorry to be such a burden to you*, in the hopes that your loved one will reassure you that you're not a burden, that you're loved, and that yes, this is a difficult time, but we'll get through it. On the face of it, this seems like an okay outcome, doesn't it? But do you see anything wrong with this picture? When you ask your loved one for reassurance about not being a burden, what are you doing? For all intents and purposes, you are asking them to do the heavy lifting of assuaging the machinations of your mind, which possibly does what? That's right, it possibly increases their sense of burden or maybe even creates one that wasn't there before.

This is where you start to see the drawback of struggling against your thoughts and trying to rid yourself of them. With experiential avoidance, you often end up causing the exact opposite effect you were looking for in the first place. You may get a momentary sense of relief, but what does it cost you?

So, what options do you have? Instead of working to rid yourself of that thought, what if you simply observe the fact that you're having it and allow it to exist without judgment or struggle? That would almost surely lead to feelings of discomfort and maybe even more unpleasant thoughts, but it also gives you the opportunity to do something else with your time and your energy rather than struggle with that distressing thought. In this process of defusion, you're engaged less with the thought itself and more with the observation of the process, thus allowing you to make better decisions about whether or not to engage with a particular thought.

Right or Wrong, It Doesn't Matter

It's important to note here that in the process of defusion, we're not really concerned with the "rightness" or "wrongness" of the thought. This is where ACT tends to differ from CBT. We're not really concerned with whether or not you actually are a burden to your family. If we argue the rationality or irrationality of the thought, that's just more struggling to vanquish it and more seeking reassurance that it isn't true. It's a different form of the same battle and still pulls us away from doing what might really matter to us. In ACT, truth lies in *function*. In regard to any thought you may have at any time, all you need to ask yourself to determine if you should engage with the thought or defuse from it is whether or not engaging with the thought will serve as a functional way of moving you towards what you value (more on this in Chapter 7) or away from it. *Is this thought useful?* If it moves you closer, then by all means, engage away! If, however, you observe that engaging with this thought interferes with leading your values-driven life, then defusion is your answer.

To return to our example regarding the thought of being a burden to your family, what would defusion look like in that circumstance? Rather than struggling with getting rid of that thought and asking your loved ones to reassure you, try this alternative:

- Observe the fact that you're having a thought.
- Name it. *I'm having a thought that I'm a burden to my family.* Better yet, *I **notice** that I'm having a thought about being a burden to my family.*
- Remember that this thought is merely a symbolic representation. Identify the connection (relational frame) you've made between your illness and your family.
- Decide what to do about that symbolic representation. If you struggle against the premise of that connection (for example, seek reassurance), that's how you expend your energy. If you simply recognize that the connection is only symbolic and need not dominate your experience of the present moment, then you give yourself the opportunity to defuse from the thought and respond with flexibility.

Rather than burdening your family with the task of reassuring you that you're not a burden, what else could you do? This varies greatly because everyone's values are different. But it's safe to assume that if you worry about being a burden to your family, you value your family. So, focus on ways to move towards what you value. You could ask your family members how they're doing, then listen to the events of their lives and their feelings.

Engage with THEM, not your thoughts about being a burden to them. Being fused with your thoughts and acting to extinguish those thoughts only adds to your problem. But being able to simply observe your thought process and respond flexibly in the moment creates an opportunity to engage in a values-driven activity that enhances your life as well as the lives of your loved ones—they also get to engage with you in a non-illness centered way.

Note that in this scenario, nothing about whether or not a burden actually exists came into play. We're not really interested in learning "the truth" about that because the only truth that matters is the *functional truth*. Fusion typically leads to a lack of functional behavior, and defusion offers you the best chance at being more functional. It's really all about what works in terms of your values.

Easier Said Than Done?

My guess is that most of you are thinking, *well, that's great, but how am I supposed to do all of that?* It's a valid question, but as I mentioned, ACT is all about doing. Defusion is a skill, just like all of the core processes of ACT. With practice, anyone can learn to do it, and practice is essential. For the remainder of this chapter, I'm going to present you with some classic ACT metaphors and exercises, some tailored to Lyme, designed to help you better understand and engage with defusion.

ACT in Metaphors and Exercises

Each of the chapters on the core processes of ACT has several metaphors and exercises to help you increase your ACT skills and abilities. Many of these metaphors and exercises are standards in the ACT literature. Others I've created and use specifically with clients who have Lyme and chronic illness. Regardless, an exhaustive list of every metaphor and technique is well beyond the scope of this book, so I strongly encourage you to explore others. You can find them by referring to the list of resources and the references at the back of the book. The metaphors and exercises below should serve as an excellent foundation for getting started with creating separation between your thinking self and your observing self.

The Basics

The first thing you can do to help facilitate defusion is to start using separatist language. For example, when having the thought *I am a burden to my family*, re-state that to something like *I am having a thought that I am a burden to my family* or even better *I notice that I am having a thought that I am a burden to my family*. Using phrases like *I notice, I observe,* or *I can see that* will help to create some separation from your thinking mind. Treat your mind as a separate entity from yourself to facilitate that process. Use phrases like *my mind is telling me that* or *I don't have to listen to my mind right now*. You can even thank your mind for making you aware of certain things but tell it that you don't want to attend to that right now because it's not that important to you (Hayes et al, 1999).

You can also do simple things like write your recurrent distressing thoughts down on index cards and carry them around with you (Hayes et al, 1999). Treat those cards as if they are your thoughts and experiences. Simply carry them around with you while you're doing other values-driven activities. Distressing thoughts can coexist with values-driven action and this will help to drive that point home.

It's not always easy to identify difficult or distressing thoughts. A good way to get at the root of this is to ask yourself if this story seems familiar or old. If you can classify something as the same old story—*I'm not good enough, people don't like me, I'm too sick to be any good to anyone, I can't do anything anymore*—then this is a pretty good indicator that this thought is worthy of defusion (Hayes et al, 1999). You have a choice as to whether or not you buy into the same old story as well as whether or not you write a new one. Don't be afraid to get creative or make your own statements or metaphors to help you increase your defusion skills. Chances are the ones you come up with will resonate much more than anything I can pass along to you. Some more complex and colorful metaphors are described below.

Your Thoughts Are Like a Menu—Pick the One You Want

Human thoughts are often compared to computer commands, so try treating your thoughts like a drop-down menu on your computer. You don't have any control over what items show up on the menu, but you do get to choose which option to click on. That choice is based on what actions you want your computer to do. You don't spend any time trying to get rid of the other menu options—you just let them be there and exist while you choose the one that matters to you the most and will get you where you want to go.

You can do the same thing with your thoughts. At any given point in time, you probably have several different thoughts running through your mind. *I'm unlovable* is right next to *I love my family*. *I can't do what I used to do* is near *I value my health*. Use the "drop-down menu" to pick the thoughts you engage with based on your valued outcome. Let the others exist and have minimal impact on your life, because they don't have to have an impact if you don't engage with them.

Similarly, when you go to a restaurant, you don't write the menu, just like you don't control your thoughts. You look over the menu and pick what you want, letting the other menu items exist as they are. You don't contact the chef and demand to have an item removed because you don't like it. You don't negotiate with the waitstaff to remove an item or rename a sandwich. You simply let the menu exist and engage with the items that you value (possibly based on health, taste, hunger, budget). Treat your thoughts the same way. You don't have to buy into every thought you have in the same way that you don't have to buy every item on a menu at a restaurant.

Getting Hooked

A less technical phrase that's often used to describe what happens when we're fused with our thinking is "getting hooked" (Whitney, 2013, in Stoddard and Afari, 2014). This metaphor comes from fly fishing. Really good fly fishers tie realistic flies and manipulate their movements on the water's surface so well that the fish can't distinguish the actual flies from the bait. The trout buys that the fly is real, bites, and gets hooked.

Your mind can be like a skilled fly fisher. Your thoughts are nothing more than sophisticated flies designed so you will take the bait and bite, getting hooked. Then the more you struggle, the more you're behaving in ways that pull the hook in further and keep you on the line. However, your mind can only tie flies on barbless hooks. It feels like you can't escape, but if you pause from the struggle and just spit the hook out—you're free. Your mind is constantly tempting you with excellent bait, but you don't have to take it. Even if you do, you don't have to continue on the ride. You can stop and spit out the hook at any time.

Passengers on the Bus

This classic ACT metaphor will help you tap into the process of defusion. It is traditionally used as an acceptance exercise (Hayes et al, 1999), but I find it works for defusion as well. Imagine you're a bus driver. You're expected to keep your route and arrive at your stops on time. At each stop, passengers get on and off the bus. Some passengers are nice and friendly, others are neutral, and some are downright nasty and mean. They yell things at you, impugning your competence as a driver. Maybe they're smelly or just plain unwanted, unwelcome, and make you feel very uncomfortable and distressed. As the bus driver, what can you do? The nasty passengers paid their fare just like the nice ones did. They're not threatening to cause you or anyone else any harm, so it's not a safety issue. If you stop the bus and argue with them or try to throw them off, they'll probably refuse to go. They have a right to public transportation. The more you fight and argue, the later you'll be in keeping to your route.

If, however, you just keep driving, letting the nasty passengers take the ride, you get to keep your schedule (and your job). And guess what? At some point, the nasty passenger will get off the bus. Thoughts, like bus passengers, come and go—the happy ones and the distressing ones all get on and off the bus. If you allow that process to happen while you keep driving the bus, you end up better off than if you stopped everything and fought or struggled with the nasty passengers.

The "Silly" Ones

ACT-ers tend to be a creative and playful bunch. If this is something that resonates with you, then you might enjoy some of the techniques described in this section. They aren't for everyone, but nothing is, so that's okay. There are several techniques that are used to enhance defusion that many would consider to be "silly" or lacking in seriousness, but a lot of defusion is exactly about not taking your thoughts too seriously, so tapping into some of that silliness can be very helpful.

Repeating thoughts to yourself over and over again tends to take some of the weightiness out of them (Titchener, 1916). Another technique is to sing your distressing thoughts to various tunes—childhood songs work well (Hayes et al, 1999). Anything from "Happy Birthday" and "Row, Row, Row Your Boat" to various nursery rhymes and songs can help you to take your uncomfortable thoughts less seriously. It's very hard to be distressed or upset or over-engaged with a thought when you're singing it to the tune of "Mary Had a Little Lamb." There are several smartphone apps that will turn your voice recording into a song, which can also be helpful.

Try challenging yourself to differentiate your thoughts from your beliefs. Treat your thoughts like bullies and remind yourself that YOU are in charge, not your mind. If you've ever been bullied or teased, think about how damaging it would be to just believe everything a bully said to you. Then think about what you would want to say to that bully (or maybe even said). Treat your mind the same way when it's feeding you nonsense that pulls you away from your values. Say to your mind what you would say to that bully—feel free to use colorful language if it helps!

You can also use silly voices, like those of your favorite cartoon characters, to say your thoughts (Stern, 2013, in Stoddard and Afari, 2014). Sounding it out also helps, which involves saying your distressing or uncomfortable thoughts very, very slowly—almost painfully slowly—to the point where you become bored with the thought itself and it loses its weight. *I...am...not... good...enou...oh, forget it.*

Although some of these ideas may seem simple, silly, or maybe even offensive to you, I encourage you to at least try them. I don't expect every technique to help every person, but you won't know what works for you and what doesn't if you don't try them. If you find yourself having the thought that these "silly ones" are not for you, challenge yourself to defuse from that thought and try them anyway. These techniques don't take a lot of effort, and you might find yourself laughing about what you thought were dire or devastating thoughts. When that happens, you can be assured that you've accomplished successful defusion!

The Mindful Ones

Mindfulness, as a central process of ACT, shows itself in all core processes, so being mindful can be very helpful in the defusion process (Hayes et al, 2012). If you commit to openness, to asking yourself if the distressing content of a thought is acceptable or not and then commit to being open to experiencing that discomfort, you're less likely to be fused with the thought and thus less likely to have it guide your behavior. Similarly, if you engage in open mindfulness—watching your thoughts as external objects without any specific use and without being involved with them—you facilitate the separation you're seeking between your thinking and observing selves. You can also physicalize your thoughts—give them some sort of imaginary form during a mindfulness exercise (you'll see some of this in Chapter 4). If your thoughts have a structure, they become less diffuse and ethereal, thus less threatening.

The Experiential Ones

Experiential-based defusion exercises are also very helpful (Hayes et al, 2012). If you're encountering a difficult or uncomfortable thought, seek out more material. Step right into the discomfort and see what happens. This is critical in dealing with anxiety. Inevitably, as people step into their anxiety and immerse themselves in activities that terrify them, they eventually become less scared. Remind yourself that thoughts are not causes—they're just thoughts—and that it's possible to think something and do something else. I promise, you pull that off every day of your life. Have you ever thought, *ugh, I can't stand that person*, but were polite and civil anyway? You acted in a way that was inconsistent with what you were thinking. That's defusion! Whenever you do something that's not dictated by your thoughts (*I dislike her*) but by your values (*I treat others well*), this is movement in the right direction.

You can also simply acknowledge that your thought is correct—concede the argument and focus on action. *My mind is telling me that I'm a burden to my family. Fine, mind, you're right, but what am I going to do about it?* Giving up the struggle (much like letting go of the rope in a tug of war) frees you up to focus on *doing* what matters rather than continuing to struggle with your mind. You can choose to be right or choose to live fully. Given the choice in any situation, what's your preference? If you refuse to argue and use "you're right" as a cue to action, you increase the likelihood that you'll move forward.

All of these defusion tools are designed to get you to live your life as fully as possible rather than waiting until you are "better" or "fixed." This process can happen right now, in this moment, no matter how distressed or sick you might feel. This is another exercise that might help. If you have a trusted friend, family member, or a therapist, try "taking your mind for a walk." You can also do this on your own with a tape recorder. Walk around the room and have your friend, therapist, or your recorded voice repeat your distressing and troubling thoughts over and over while you're doing other things. This reinforces the reality that you can be functional and do things while distressing or uncomfortable thoughts are rattling around in your head.

A Mindfulness Defusion Exercise: Dandelions in the Wind

This is a variation of a rather famous metaphor called "Leaves on a Stream" (Hayes et al, 1999). It was further utilized by Russ Harris (2009), a psychiatrist based in New Zealand and an icon in the ACT movement. "Leaves on a Stream" is widely available in many published works and in various places online. It was created as an exercise for defusion. This is a version I frequently use that I think creates a nice platform for dealing with difficult thoughts:

> *Sit in a comfortable position and either close your eyes or rest them gently on a fixed spot in the room. Take several slow, mindful breaths, paying close attention to the sensation of the air moving in and out of your lungs. After a few moments, visualize yourself*

sitting in a peaceful field or country meadow. The dandelions are going to seed, and a gentle wind is blowing. As the breeze flows, it carries the wispy dandelion seeds along with it. For the next few minutes, imagine each thought that enters your mind as one of those dandelion seeds. Let the breeze carry it along its current, moving lightly in the air. Do this with each thought—pleasurable, painful, or neutral. Even if you have joyous or enthusiastic thoughts, imagine they are just dandelion wisps and let them float by. If your thoughts momentarily stop, continue to watch the wisps float on by in the breeze. Sooner or later, your thoughts will start up again. Allow the breeze to blow at its own pace. Don't try to speed it up and rush your thoughts along. You're not trying to rush the dandelion seeds or "get rid" of your thoughts. You're simply allowing them to come and go at their own pace. If your mind says, this is dumb, I'm bored, *or* I'm not doing this right, *place those thoughts on the dandelion wisps too. Let them float away in the breeze. If a dandelion hovers or gets stuck, allow it to hang around until it passes by with the breeze. If the thought comes up again, watch it pass by another time. If a difficult or painful feeling arises, simply acknowledge it. Say to yourself,* I notice myself having a feeling of boredom/impatience/frustration. *See those thoughts as dandelions and allow them to float along. From time to time, your thoughts may hook you and distract you from being fully present in this exercise. This is normal. As soon as you realize that you've become sidetracked, gently bring your attention back to the visualization exercise.*

This exercise reinforces several aspects of the ACT process. It helps you stay grounded in the present (or be mindful), which is almost always a good thing. It provides a nice metaphor that you can carry with you even when you're not engaged in the actual mindfulness exercise. If you practice this enough, you will get to the point where you can pretty easily visualize putting difficult or uncomfortable thoughts on a dandelion tuft and letting them blow away with the breeze without judgment or struggle. You can do the same with any of the metaphors mentioned previously. Whether your thoughts are silly songs, goofy characters, passengers on the bus, slow talkers, or bullies on the playground, the more you use the techniques and create different relational frames, the greater the distance between your thinking self and your observing self. This separation creates more room for psychological flexibility, which is the goal.

Boat on the Water

A similar exercise to "Leaves on the Stream" or "Dandelions in the Wind" is "Boat on the Water" (Bryan, 2013, in Stoddard and Afari, 2014). Rather than placing thoughts on objects and watching them float away, you experience the rise and fall of thoughts as if you were on a boat.

> Close your eyes and imagine you're on a boat in the ocean. Engage all of your senses as you float along. Smell the ocean air. Feel the sun on your skin. Picture the horizon meeting the ocean. Feel the boat swaying beneath you. Gentle waves begin to hit the boat. You feel it rise and fall as you hear each small wave lap against the hull. Almost as soon as you realize a wave has come, it passes. It's not long before another comes along. Sometimes the waves come quickly and powerfully, then pass. Sometimes the waves seem so big they're all you can see, until they too pass. As the waves continuously go past you—some big, some small—feel each one. And as you do, try to notice any thoughts or feelings that arise as well. As you notice these internal experiences, see if you can just ride the waves, allowing the thoughts and feelings to rise and fall, come and go. Stay on the boat, and if you get swept overboard into the water, simply recognize that this has happened, climb back in the boat, and continue to ride the waves.

This exercise helps you to tap into the transient rise and fall of difficult thoughts and emotions. You can't control your thoughts any more easily than you can control the waves of the ocean. But you can allow the waves to happen, to come and go, as they will do.

Caveats and Pitfalls

Virtually all of the ACT processes carry with them the risk of being misapplied, misunderstood, or generally misused. I'll take a few moments in each chapter to address some of these pitfalls. Additionally, I'll address them more globally in Chapter 9.

It's important to remember that ACT isn't about trying to ignore every thought you have. Indeed, ACT doesn't want you to ignore any of your thoughts, because it's really not possible. Instead, defusion is about recognizing your thoughts for what they are—connected symbolic representations (relational frames) based on the experiences of your life. There is no need to judge them or struggle against them. In fact, the more you do either of those things, the worse things will tend to get for you. You will certainly have thoughts that need to be attended to, that will help you solve problems and move you in valued directions in your life. Your mind is not evil, and it's not out to get you, but it's not perfect either. Sometimes it will feed you information that isn't particularly helpful. Remember, thoughts are not good or evil, right or wrong, healthy or unhealthy—they just are. Our main concern is whether or not engaging with a particular thought, at a given point in time, in a given context, will serve the function of moving your life forward. That's it.

Our job is simply to create enough separation between our thinking selves and our observing selves so we're not beholden to our thought processes and we can have enough psychological flexibility to act in ways that are in accordance with what we value and what is truly important to us. Right now, in this moment, you can't control the fact that you're sick, nor can you control the fact that you have a litany of distressing, uncomfortable, unpleasant, true or untrue, healthy or unhealthy, good or bad, right or wrong thoughts knocking around in your mind at any given point in time. The only question you have to answer in terms of what thought to engage with is whether or not that engagement moves you towards what you value and what is really important to you. Anything else is a waste of your time and energy; and you need every bit of that you can spare.

Thoughts, of course, are only part of the puzzle. Emotions come right along with them and as tricky as your mind can be, your emotions can be even trickier and more difficult to co-exist with. This brings us to our second core process of ACT, Acceptance.

Chapter 4

The Paradox of Acceptance

Acceptance doesn't mean resignation; it means understanding that something is what it is and that there's got to be a way through it.
Michael J. Fox

What Is Acceptance?

Of all the concepts in ACT, I've found that acceptance is the one people struggle with the most. It's also the one that's most likely to be misunderstood. As such, acceptance can be a hard sell, especially when dealing with chronic illness. As mentioned earlier, some of the suggestions and approaches in this book may seem counterintuitive and difficult. This chapter is the most likely place for you to have some of those reactions. So, let me reiterate my request that you keep reading and try to remain open to what acceptance is all about. If you approach this chapter with an open mind and give it a chance, it could have a profound impact on your life. Not only is acceptance one of the most widely misunderstood concepts and processes in ACT, it is arguably the most important and may just hold the key to living a better life than you're living right now.

Common Misunderstanding about Acceptance

The quote at the beginning of this chapter from Michael J. Fox, who lives with Parkinson's disease, is there for a reason. Acceptance does not mean giving up. I'll say that again, because it's that important. *Acceptance does not mean giving up.* It's not about "pulling yourself up by your bootstraps" and moving on, or "sucking it up" and merely tolerating unpleasant or difficult emotions or circumstances in your life. Most of you have probably already heard that kind of advice, and I'm guessing you didn't find it very helpful. In fact, it wouldn't surprise me if you were pretty put off by it or if it made you angry.

Acceptance is also not approval of what's happening, agreeing with it, liking it, or judging it as positive. No one is asking you to feel great about being sick or think that it's the best thing that's ever happened to you. People often assume that the process of accepting something means you are inherently approving of it or that it must become a "good thing" in your life, but that could not be further from the truth. The good news is that those "approaches" or misconceptions completely miss the core concept of what acceptance in ACT is really all about.

Acceptance in ACT

Acceptance has an ancient history rooted in Eastern philosophy and religion. Many modern psychotherapy approaches have embraced varying definitions of acceptance as core parts of their therapeutic models. In ACT, acceptance is defined as "the voluntary adoption of an intentionally open, receptive, flexible, and non-judgmental posture with respect to moment-to-moment experience" (Hayes et al, 2012, p. 272). Another way of looking at acceptance is being open to the full range of experiences that your life has to offer, both pleasant and unpleasant, and having a willingness and flexibility to live your life while embracing the reality that there will be difficulty and pain as well as happiness, joy, and everything in between.

This is a somewhat foreign concept in our culture because we are constantly sold the idea that we are supposed to be happy or feeling great all the time, and if we're not then something is wrong with us. The reality is that life inherently involves difficulty and pain—there is no avoiding it. The only real question is what you decide to do with that pain and difficulty when you're experiencing it.

These are powerful and important concepts that may be hard to wrap your head around if your life has been sidelined by a debilitating disease. The idea of "voluntarily adopting an intentionally open and non-judgmental posture" regarding your illness—the very thing that has turned your life upside down, perhaps put you out of work, maybe caused difficulty in your relationships with your friends and family—seems counterintuitive at best and downright ridiculous or insulting at worst. Admittedly, acceptance in the context of chronic illness seems a bit more complicated than in other situations, so let's take a step back to make sure we understand the basic concepts of acceptance first. A non-chronic illness case example might help to introduce this core process at work.

Non-Chronic Illness Case Example: Emily

Emily is a 25-year-old single woman who suffers from social anxiety. She has a supportive family, a decent job, and lots of close friends. But she has tremendous difficulty interacting with people she doesn't know, especially men. When she finds herself in these situations, she becomes very anxious and tongue-tied. As a result, she frequently avoids going out to public places with friends or talking with men she might be interested in dating. If she's out and decides that she wants to take a risk and talk to someone, especially a man, she will invariably have a few drinks to "take the edge off" before doing so. Over time, Emily's withdrawal from social situations and use of alcohol to cope with her anxiety led her to become more and more isolated, and her drinking increased to the point where she was frequently doing it by herself.

Eventually, she came to recognize that alcohol was just another form of escape and avoidance of her anxiety. She realized that if she were to really pursue what mattered to her—having a meaningful romantic relationship—she would have to consciously choose to be anxious in the process of doing so. Her attempts to avoid the anxiety were actually keeping her from doing what really mattered because she either avoided the process altogether or was too affected by alcohol to genuinely experience anything meaningful. When she chose to openly and willingly accept her anxiety, it became less dangerous and powerful and thus had less influence over her life. It did not go away, but she managed to change her relationship with it and become more social in the process.

Emily and Experiential Avoidance

Emily's situation perfectly illustrates the concept of experiential avoidance. This phenomenon "occurs when a person is unwilling to remain in contact with particular private experiences (bodily sensations, emotions, thoughts, memories, behavioral predispositions) and takes steps to alter the form, frequency, or situational sensitivity of these experiences even though doing so is not immediately necessary" (Hayes et al, 2012, pp. 72–3). Emily was avoiding her social anxiety by eliminating (or altering with alcohol) the social experiences that triggered her symptoms.

In other words, experiential avoidance is deliberately not participating in certain activities in the futile attempt to prevent the experience of unpleasant emotions, sensations, or difficult circumstances in our lives. I use the word futile quite purposely here because, while experiential avoidance may be an effective strategy for avoiding unpleasant emotions in the short term (Emily usually felt relief after deciding not to do something social), in the long term it's simply impossible to live a life free of unpleasant emotional experiences. It just isn't human. While Emily experienced short-term relief by not going to a party or by drinking too much while she was there, she closed herself off to what she really valued—genuine human contact—because it was painful to her.

The idea behind acceptance is that if you're willing to open yourself up to the full range of human experiences, your life is no longer hindered by experiential avoidance. You get to do what's really important to you, regardless of how you might feel.

The Paradox of Acceptance

Acceptance versus Experiential Avoidance

The real cause of suffering in people's lives is not the pain they experience (illness, anxiety, depression, loneliness, insecurity, etc.) but their attempts to avoid that pain. In Emily's case, she avoided social situations or drank so she could tolerate them. In either scenario, she ultimately lost because she did not extinguish her anxiety (it kept coming back, as it tends to do), and she did not get what she really wanted — meaningful social interactions.

If Emily decided to go to the party and not drink, I'm not saying this would be an easy experience for her. She would likely have a significant amount of anxiety, maybe even panic, and this is extremely unpleasant, hence the pull towards experiential avoidance. However, if she allows herself to experience this emotional pain and changes her relationship with it in service of something that is worthwhile to her (for example, genuine human contact) then it makes sense to do so. The reward of having a meaningful experience is almost always worth the risk of experiencing difficult emotions.

I would never ask anyone to put themselves in a painful situation if it's not moving them in a desired direction in their life (more on this in Chapter 7), and you shouldn't ask this of yourself either. Experiencing pain in service of what you value is a fundamental necessity and truism of human existence. It's our attempts to avoid experiencing this pain that lead to suffering. Pain is a fundamental state of being human, but suffering is a choice that depends entirely on how we approach the pain in our lives.

In other words, if we remain open to experiencing all that life has to offer (or sometimes throws at us) no matter how difficult and painful it might be, we have a much better chance at moving our lives in directions that are meaningful to us. The more we try not to feel, the more our lives get stuck. Much like we discussed in Chapter 3 about how futile it is to try not to think something, it is equally futile to try not to feel something. When you spend your life in service of experiential avoidance (trying not to feel), you really don't get anywhere and it usually leads to suffering.

Take a Ride on a Balloon

The experience of acceptance is a lot like flying in a hot-air balloon. They both offer the potential of something beautiful—seeing the world in a totally different and fantastic way that's not easily available to you on a day-to-day basis. However, ballooning is also fraught with danger. While doing it with an experienced professional is a pretty safe activity, the fact of the matter is that you're high up in the air, subject to weather events, mechanical failure, and other flying objects. Anything could go wrong. But if you want the beautiful vistas, you have to *willingly choose* to accept the risk (as evidenced by the waiver you will most likely have to sign). If you choose not to accept the risk, you don't get to experience all the beauty and joy the balloon ride has to offer. This mirrors the reality of life—if you don't accept that awful things can and sometimes will happen, your life will be less full, less meaningful, and less vital. It may be "safer," but at what cost?

Moreover, if you want to go anywhere in a balloon, you need to burn the fuel (feel the emotions). This is what fills the balloon and gives it lift. If you turn off the fuel (try to stop feeling the emotions) you'll be grounded, unable to go anywhere. But if you open up the flame and let the fuel burn—if you allow yourself to experience your emotions—the balloon (and your life) gets bigger and lighter. The next thing you know, you're on your way, which is what you wanted in the first place. Interestingly enough, no matter how much fuel you burn or how hot the air gets, hot-air balloons don't burst. The result of burning the fuel (again, feeling the emotions) only allows you to fly higher. The hot air never becomes bigger than the balloon itself, just as your emotions can never become bigger than you are, even though most of us are terrified of being overwhelmed by our emotions.

You may have little control over where the wind takes you, but it's balloonist tradition to fly wherever, land wherever, and simply enjoy the journey for its own sake. Our own lives do not have to be quite so directionless and subject to the changing winds, but we all have times where attempting to control the direction or events of our lives takes a whole lot of effort but has very little effect. ACT in general and acceptance specifically are much more about letting go and embracing the journey wherever it may take us, as long as that journey is truly important to us.

Climbing Mountains

I can give you another example related to my personal experience. I love to climb mountains—big mountains. I've been doing it for the last 10 plus years with my best friend from childhood. Once a year we get together and take a climbing trip. If you've ever done any kind of physical activity like this, you come to understand pretty quickly that it's a grueling endeavor. You're exerting yourself very intensely with less atmospheric oxygen in sometimes bitter cold and high winds, sleeping (if you can) in very uncomfortable tents on rocks or glaciers or anything else that's definitely not your mattress at home. Moreover, in order to be ready to do something like this, you have to be in reasonably good physical condition, which involves lots of training all year round, being constantly vigilant about your weight and nutrition, investing time in regular exercise, etc. In short, it takes a lot of time, hard work, and even pain to get to the top. This is so much the case that there is an old saying in mountaineering that goes something like this: "Mountaineering is like hitting yourself in the head with a hammer. It feels great once you stop." There is a lot of truth in that. I have exerted myself to the point of exhaustion and pain in service of this activity more times than I care to count.

All of which begs the question, why would I put myself through all of this? Why not just vacation at a beach and relax?

There are several answers to this question, for me anyway. The views, obviously, are beautiful. I've seen sights that most people will never see and been places where most people will never go. I've shared amazing experiences with my best friend and bonded with him in a way that is fundamentally different and deeper than you can bond with someone while lying on a beach (not that I have anything against beach vacations!). It motivates me to stay in shape and be as healthy as I can because I can't do what I love if I'm not physically capable. It helps me to achieve a level of deep concentration and focus that I don't easily attain on a daily basis with family, clients, students, colleagues, friends, etc. It brings me closer to nature and helps me feel more connected with myself and the world I live in. In short, I love it, so I do what I have to do because the pain is in service of what I truly value in my life.

The Reward of Acceptance

In order for me to do what I love, what's really important to me, I have to accept that there are unpleasant aspects to that pursuit. I don't really like going outside for a run in the middle of winter when it is freezing cold. But if I want to experience all of the things that are important to me, I have to be okay with "hitting myself in the head with a hammer" from time to time, so to speak. If I decide to avoid all of the unpleasantness that comes with climbing mountains, then I lose all of the pleasure and joy as well. They are two sides of the same coin. I can either keep the whole coin or throw it all away. Ironically enough, throwing away the coin wouldn't make me immune to suffering, just as staying home or drinking too much didn't make Emily immune to suffering either. How fulfilled have you been in your life when you're not moving towards what's important to you?

As humans beings we're meant to experience a broad range of emotions, from very painful and unpleasant to very pleasurable and joyful. It's human nature to try to avoid painful experiences.

But when this keeps us from engaging in meaningful activities in our lives, we're engaging in experiential avoidance and we get stuck. However, if we open ourselves up to experiencing the full range of human emotions, however unpleasant, we free ourselves to move towards what is really important to us. This is the reward of acceptance.

Acceptance in Chronic Illness: Choice versus Control

Now that you have the basic idea about acceptance and its role in our lives, you may wonder how to apply it to your illness (and not Emily's social anxiety or my mountains). You're probably saying to yourself that if I want to go on a balloon ride or climb a mountain, it's all well and good to accept the painful aspects because it's my choice to do those things or not do them. You, however, did not choose to be sick and certainly can't just decide to not be sick anymore, so how does any of this apply to what you're going through? This is a fabulous question that highlights another misconception about acceptance, which has to do with choice and control.

Many people labor under the notion that acceptance is easy when you have a choice regarding what you do, but what about when things are thrust upon you, things over which you have no control? Doesn't acceptance mean that whatever happens, happens? We're just supposed to cede all control of our lives to the fates? Having a chronic illness puts you at a higher risk of adopting this position, but it could not be further from the truth. In fact, acceptance is at its greatest importance exactly when we're dealing with situations that are beyond our control.

In their wonderful book *Things Might Go Terribly, Horribly Wrong* (2010), Kelly Wilson (an ACT founder) and Troy DuFrene describe a classic and powerful example of a man who accepted his horrific circumstances and led a meaningful existence despite them. Viktor Frankl was a psychiatrist who was sent to several concentration camps during World War II where he was surrounded by unspeakable horrors and where his entire family, save his sister, died. Being the physician that he was, he did all he could to tend to the health and well-being of those suffering and dying around him. And he found meaning in this activity. When he was given the opportunity to move to a rest camp—to effectively alleviate much of his own suffering—he chose to stay in the concentration camp and continue to make his rounds and help those to whom he was tending. In this situation of tremendous pain and horror that was thrust upon him and over which he had no control, he found a way to live meaningfully amidst his pain. So meaningfully, in fact, that when he had the opportunity to ease his own pain, to leave that horrible place, he chose to continue doing what was truly important to him. He chose to say "yes" to living in a concentration camp.

Frankl, of course, went on to write about his experience in his classic book *Man's Search for Meaning*. Not surprisingly, he also became the founder of Logotherapy, a form of existential psychotherapy that emphasizes the importance of seeking meaning in life, no matter what the circumstances. Frankl had no choice about the origin of his pain. He could not easily solve his problems. But, by tapping into the meaning in his life, by changing his relationship to his pain and suffering, he transformed himself and helped countless others in the process. Frankl was an extraordinary human being living under extraordinary circumstances in extraordinary times, *but so are you*. If Frankl found a way to do it, you can too.

We Are Problem-Solving Machines

Human beings are problem-solving machines. We see or feel something wrong and we put all of our impressive brain power into making that problem go away or get better as quickly as possible. Inherently, of course, this isn't a bad thing. It's a wonderful gift we have that has made our world a far better and more comfortable place to be. However, problem solving is really only effective when we're dealing with solvable problems. Many issues we struggle with in our lives, such as chronic illness, are not solvable problems, at least not in an immediate sense. So, the real distinguishing characteristic here is being able to figure out what aspects of your life you have some control over and what aspects you do not. For example, if you walk down a dark alley late at night and you see a group of unsavory characters with weapons and menacing looks on their faces at the other end of the alley, I would never recommend that you "accept your path," walk down the alley, and remain open to the experience of getting mugged. I would wholeheartedly recommend that you turn around and head for a well-lit area with lots of other people around. That's a solvable problem.

But what happens when the problem isn't so easily solved? What happens if you're so tired or in so much pain that you can't get out of bed or your brain is so foggy that you can't think straight? What happens when you try to seek treatment but get caught in the quagmire of a medical debate that has hindered your doctor's ability to help you? What happens when your spouse is doing all of the work with the kids and the house because your joints hurt so much that you can't walk down the driveway, let alone grocery shop or go to work? You chose none of this, and all you really want is for it to go away. So, your natural instinct is to engage with the problem-solving machine and work really hard at finding a solution. Unfortunately, this isn't as easy as turning around in the alley. When you can't immediately solve these problems, where does it leave you? Instead, you have to figure out how to live your life the best way that you can under the circumstances, however difficult that may seem.

Chronic Illness + Problem Solving = Experiential Avoidance

I don't mean to sound ominous here, but the fundamental reality is that people with chronic illnesses don't have easily solvable problems. If they did, they wouldn't be ill anymore. I also don't mean to dismiss problem solving altogether. Of course, if you're ill, you should seek all the medical help you can get. Obtain second, third, fourth, and fifth opinions if necessary. Assuming that your health and well-being are important to you, you should do whatever's necessary to maintain and enhance them as much as possible.

Unfortunately, when dealing with chronic illness, especially Lyme disease, it's not that simple. All of this takes time, effort, and often money. Even under the best of circumstances, sometimes all the medical help in the world will not bring you back to your previous level of functioning or have you feeling your best in this moment. This may leave you feeling deeply sad, angry, frustrated, or hopeless, among many other emotions. If your intent is to "solve" your problem so you don't have to feel those emotions anymore, to make the unpleasantness go away, you're engaging in experiential avoidance, and this will likely not improve your life. In fact, it will probably get you stuck.

A Different Path: Acceptance

Acceptance isn't about being okay with being sick, it's about being open to your unique, internal, private experience of being sick. If you stop pouring all of your energy into making the pain and the emotions go away, is it possible that you just might create enough wiggle room to move towards something more rewarding and more valuable in your life? Maybe, if you put the energy that you use trying not to *feel* (angry or sad or whatever) into your kids, your partner, your friends, a hobby—anything that really matters—this might just help you to have a better experience in the moment. You might not be able to do this to the fullest extent you'd like, but *any* movement towards what is truly important to you is movement in the right direction and energy well spent.

Will acceptance cure your symptoms? Will acceptance make the sadness or anger go away? Most likely not. But in ACT, extinguishing difficult thoughts and unpleasant feelings is almost never the goal. On the contrary, if you allow yourself to experience *all* of your feelings—if you don't invest yourself in fighting them off—then you might be able to engage in something more meaningful.

Of course, you may not be able to engage in a valued activity as well as you did before you were sick. But your comparison can't be your life prior to your illness, just as you can't compare yourself to your peers or to a younger version of yourself. You are who you are at this moment in time—a unique person with experiences that are exclusive to you. Accepting yourself as you are is a choice that can only be made in the present moment. In short, at any given point in time, regardless of how you feel, you're either doing what gives your life meaning or you're not. Even if you can't engage in those meaningful activities as well as you used to or as much as you'd like, any little bit is better than not doing them at all.

Why Acceptance Seems Counterintuitive

We're wired to make uncomfortable or "bad" thoughts and feelings go away. You perceive a threat, you experience fear, you act in a way to reduce that fear (avoid or conquer the threat), you feel safe, and you feel better. It's how we've survived all these thousands of years. But we now live in a time where every stimulus doesn't necessarily pose a life-threatening situation for us. In fact, most situations don't. But we tend to experience them internally as if they do, so our instinct is to put all of our efforts into making uncomfortable feelings go away because then we're "safe." But often, instead of trying to avoid fear, discomfort, or distress, what we really need to do is make an active choice to experience them—to be psychologically flexible enough to be in the moment and allow ourselves to experience our pain in a fundamentally different way that's free of suffering. This is the paradox of acceptance.

I recognize this may seem like a very difficult and scary thing to do. It might not even make much sense to you right now, but as mentioned in Chapter 2, experiential avoidance tends to be a byproduct of how we use language to make sense of our world. We have to remember, however, that our use of language is just that—*our* use of language. As such, it's subject to the same flaws, biases, and mistakes of any other human process. ACT seeks to help us step out of that self-imposed trap by creating some separation between our real, unique selves and what we think and feel. The real question then is how exactly do we do this?

Acceptance in Action

There are many, many different exercises for enhancing acceptance and willingness. The use of metaphors like the balloon and the mountain climber are often helpful in grasping the concepts. But ultimately, *one must engage in more experiential processes to build this skill*. It's just like anything else, the more you practice, the better you'll get at it. I've encouraged you at several points to explore other ACT resources, and I'll repeat that encouragement here.

While I'm providing you with an experiential exercise geared specifically towards helping with your experience of your illness, this doesn't mean that other ACT resources won't be useful to you. If this one works, great, try to find others that do as well. If it doesn't work, don't give up. There's probably an exercise out there for you that will.

The exercise below is adapted largely from Russ Harris's work (Harris, 2009). I'd recommend reading it through a few times to get the hang of the "script," then doing it as a full-on mindfulness exercise. You could also record yourself (or someone else) guiding you through the exercise and use the recording, if that's helpful. Either way, don't worry too much about rigidly adhering to the script. This is a guide. As long as you remain true to the overall spirit of the exercise, it doesn't matter if you miss a word or a sentence here or there. As with all mindfulness exercises, if you find yourself drifting, just gently acknowledge that and guide yourself back to the exercise.

Acceptance and Willingness Exercise: Giving It Form

For this exercise, find a comfortable place to sit or lie down and a time when you won't be interrupted or distracted. Settle into a comfortable position with your hands at your side. Close your eyes if you're comfortable doing that, or focus on a specific point in the room if that's easier for you. Take a few easy breaths. Focus on how the breath feels as it goes in and out of your body...the coolness as it goes in and the warmth as it goes out. Notice how the cushion feels against your back and your legs...the feel of the material on your hands and arms...the feeling of your clothes on your body. Just stay in this space for a few minutes, focus on your senses, what you hear, see, smell, feel on your body. If you find yourself drifting, just gently acknowledge that and come back to your sensory experiences.

Now, in a gentle and compassionate way, I invite you to focus on your illness. Bring yourself to the place of distress that is associated with your experience of Lyme disease. This may feel uncomfortable, but that's okay. Just try to notice and sit with that feeling rather than pushing it away. With each breath, feel yourself expanding around that feeling and loosening up around it. Whatever the feeling is—sadness, anger, frustration, fear, pain—just remain open to feeling it rather than running away from it or pushing it away. Just breathe into it and expand around it. As you feel that discomfort, really try to attend to the feeling itself. In what part of your body does the feeling reside? Where do you experience it, where does it feel most intense? Focus on how it feels in that part of your body. Try to imagine what kind of shape or form it might have. Does it have a color? If you were to touch it, what would it feel like?

Would it be warm or cold? Rough or smooth? Soft or hard? Notice all of these aspects of the feeling—observe them with curiosity. Touch the form of your feeling, imagine holding it in your hands, not altering or changing it, but just holding it lightly and watching it. What does it do? It may get smaller or bigger. It may pulse or move. It may feel warm or cold. Just notice and observe these things curiously. Recognize that even if the feeling gets bigger, no matter how big it gets, it doesn't get any heavier as you hold it. It doesn't consume or overtake you. It just exists, doing its thing.

Now imagine dropping it or letting it go—not throwing or pushing it away—but just dropping it or letting it go. It may stay close to you. It may drift away a little bit and then come back. But you are just noticing it, what it does, how it exists. Just attend to the feeling as it exists outside of you for a little bit. Do you notice how the feeling can be there and you can do other things? Your mind has probably drifted several times by now, so you know you can do other things while the feeling is there. Just focus on that coexistence for a bit. After some time, allow the form to come back to you, to be part of you again. But notice if your experience of it has changed at all. Not whether the feeling has changed, but how your relationship with it may be a bit different. Just sit with that experience for a bit.

When you are ready, begin to focus on your senses again—the feeling of the floor beneath your feet, the cushion, your breath moving through your lungs. Take a few more easy breaths, and just try to soak in the experience

Moving Forward with Acceptance

After "giving it form," do you notice anything different about the feeling? This exercise is designed to accomplish a couple of different things, mainly to create some separation between you and your experience of your illness. When you give it some kind of form that you can visualize, it makes it a bit easier to imagine it being outside yourself and not dominating your life quite as much. You'll note that nothing in the exercise asked you to change your illness or to change your feelings about your illness but rather to create a different perspective or relationship with those feelings. In the end of the exercise, you were asked to allow the feeling back in to your body. This was purposeful. True acceptance means to choose to receive something, and choosing to accept your illness—to coexist with it and all the feelings associated with it rather than struggle against those feelings every moment of every day—is an essential step to living a vital, meaningful life, even though you may be feeling sick. This does *not* mean that you don't fight your Lyme and do everything you can to get well. It *does* mean that you can't fight every moment of your experience with Lyme and live well while getting better.

Lyme and Chronic Illness: Unwanted Guests at the Party of Your Life

Having a chronic illness is much like having an annoying, unwanted guest at a party, a classic ACT metaphor (Hayes et al, 1999). Imagine you're throwing a party and someone in your life who's annoying, bothersome, rude, obnoxious, or just plain not fun shows up, uninvited. No matter how hard you try to close the door and keep him out, he finds a way to stick his feet in the doorway, come around back, or sneak in a window. You can't leave your own party, so what choice do you have? Fight and argue with the annoying unwanted guest? Call the police? What does that do to your experience of the party? How do your other guests, treasured friends, and family feel when a full-blown fight breaks out and the police arrive? Obviously, this won't lead to a desired outcome. So, what do you do?

Is it possible that if you choose to just engage with your friends and family, the people at the party who *really matter* to you, your experience of the annoying unwanted guest might change? Maybe he fades into the background a little bit and you're able to have a better—even if not ideal—experience at your party, despite the presence of the unwanted guest. You may not have a choice about his presence, but you DO have a choice about how you engage with him no matter how loud, annoying, or disruptive he may be. If your entire focus is on him, your experience of the party will be pretty lousy. But if you focus on the guests that matter—the guests who fill your life with meaning and vitality—well, that changes things a bit, doesn't it?

True acceptance is not merely tolerating the unwanted guest; instead you are willingly choosing not to fight his presence but rather to engage in meaningful things despite his unwanted attendance. This is an extraordinarily difficult concept to embrace when it comes to a debilitating chronic illness, but if you don't want your pain and difficult emotions regarding your Lyme to rule your life, you have to make room for them. I'm guessing that your attempts thus far to get rid of them haven't met with much success. Maybe it's time to try something a bit different? Instead of trying to banish your emotions, try allowing them to be present, unwanted as they may be, while you carry on and engage with the party in the best way you can. You may find that this approach creates the possibility of changing your experience with pain and difficult emotions.

Lessons from Paralysis to Overcome Paralysis

Many of you may still be feeling a bit hesitant about where we're going with this. The pull is really to make the unwanted and uncomfortable thoughts and feelings go away so we can feel better physically and emotionally, right? Well, in the same way the person with a panic disorder can't simply stop having panic attacks, you can't instantly cure your illness. It will take time for you to get better, which means you have to *decide how to live in this moment*. So, finding ways to coexist with it, to treat yourself with compassion, and to live your life in the best way you can even though you may have very debilitating symptoms,

The Paradox of Acceptance

is critical to your well-being.

The good news is that in addition to Dr. Frankl, there are plenty of other examples of acceptance from which to draw inspiration. As distressing as your Lyme may be, we can all agree that others also endure difficult and debilitating circumstances and find ways to lead enriching and fulfilling lives despite their symptoms. For example, there has been quite a bit of research done on spinal cord injury patients and how they recover quality of life after experiencing such a devastating and life-altering event. Much of this research was done well before ACT became a mainstream therapeutic approach.

Perhaps not surprisingly, a significant predictor of quality of life among spinal cord injury patients is acceptance. Studies consistently show that spinal cord injury patients who are less accepting of their condition experience more pain and lower quality of life (Summers et al, 1991; Weitzner et al, 2011; Henwood and Ellis, 2004). Certainly there is a period of adjustment fraught with emotional turmoil, but the patients who manage to regain their lives are those who stop railing against their own emotional and physical pain and allow themselves to be psychologically flexible. I would guess none of them are "happy" about their loss of functioning, but the ones who move on to lead rich and meaningful lives are those who recognize the necessity of accepting their circumstances, no matter how permanent, dire, or severe.

Acceptance is not just a powerful tool for recovery in spinal cord injury, but the impact of the ACT model is evident across a host of other medical conditions, including chronic pain (Dahl et al, 2005; Vowles and Thompson, 2011), epilepsy (Dahl and Lundgren, 2011), diabetes and obesity (Gregg et al, 2011), smoking cessation (Bricker, 2011), insomnia (Lundh, 2011), cancer, and terminal illness (Carlson and Halifax, 2011), among others. There is no reason that someone suffering from Lyme disease or any other chronic illness should not benefit from this approach. One just has to be willing to experience it.

Remember, as we discussed, acceptance is not giving up and just letting life happen. That would be a very passive way to exist. Acceptance is an active, conscious, and willing choice that anyone can make at any time—just as the spinal cord injury patients and Dr. Frankl did. While ACT is an acronym, the fact that it also spells a word that has meaning unto itself should not be lost on you. It is an active approach to living your life, and the acceptance piece of the model is no exception.

We Are Always Whole

Human history is replete with examples of people rising above the most horrific of circumstances to lead exemplary lives. It's a common theme in human existence, so much so that every major religion has a fundamental teaching about the necessity of accepting pain and truth in your life in order to live fully. That is not an accident. These are ancient concepts that have been lost along the way in a life led more comfortably because of advances in science and technology.

While science and technology are wonderful things, our own science of healing has gotten caught up in the "have to make it go away" syndrome. There is tremendous value in this approach for many, many conditions, which is why it's pervasive. But for some illnesses, especially chronic ones, the "make it go away" mentality is incredibly destructive. It can create a feeling of being broken, incomplete, and inadequate. In other words, if you're sick, you're not whole.

What ACT shows us, especially through acceptance, is that no matter what happens in our lives, we are *always* whole. In fact, it's the very experiences that we fear will break us that make us complete as human beings, along with all of the joy and happiness that comes from living life fully. Understanding ourselves in this manner brings us to the next core process of the ACT model: Self-As-Context.

Chapter 5

You Are When You Are: Self-As-Context

All bad qualities center round the ego. When the ego is gone, Realization results by itself. There are neither good nor bad qualities in the Self. The Self is free from all qualities. Qualities pertain to the mind only.
Ramana Maharshi

Getting Centered

As I mentioned in Chapter 2, the six core processes of ACT can be divided into three categories—open, centered, and engaged. We've covered the "open" side of the model with defusion and acceptance. Self-as-context moves us from the "open" processes in the ACT model to the "centered" processes, which also includes contact with the present moment addressed in the following chapter. This shift is significant for several reasons. First, it addresses an important aspect of the ACT approach, which is to be flexibly present and centered on your moment-to-moment experience regardless of what that experience may be. Second, you will begin to see to a greater degree how the ACT processes relate to one another and start to get a sense of how fluid the ACT approach really is. I touched on the basics of self-as-context in Chapter 2, as you may remember...you are not defined by your conceptualized self or your illness. This can be a confusing and difficult process to grasp, so I'll try to make it as easy as possible.

There are many different ways to view and discuss the concept of self. Some people refer to ideas such as self-concept, self-esteem, self-awareness, and of course there are the varying philosophical approaches to conceptualizing the self. In short, it can all become very confusing. Even within ACT, if you read different texts you may see different terms used to describe the concepts being discussed here. As such, it's important to enter this process without any preconceived notions regarding the definition of "self." Much like in the acceptance chapter, I will lay some groundwork so we can move forward on solid footing.

Perspective Taking

I think one of the easiest ways to approach self-as-context is to consider it in terms of perspective taking. It's not so much an idea but more of a constant process or lens through which we view the world and our experience of it. The goal is to take a flexible approach to our moment-to-moment experiences, free of interference from the mind, or our history, or the stories we've told ourselves for probably many years. The idea behind self-as-context is to create a place where we can willingly and flexibly observe our lives rather than run from discomfort, difficult feelings, or problematic situations. Much like defusion is the process of noticing our thoughts and just allowing them to happen, self-as-context allows us to notice the events of our lives and separate them from our conceptions of what any of it means related to our history and the content of our lives. In other words, it helps to "lighten the load."

The Lighthouse

A good metaphor might help at this point, so let's give it a try and see where it takes us. This is another adaption of one of Russ Harris's metaphors to describe self-as-context (Harris, 2009). Think of yourself as a lighthouse operator on a proverbial dark and stormy night. As you cast your light over the sea and the shoreline, you see rocks, waves, and ships. The things illuminated by the beam represent your concept of who you are—the content of your life—healthy or ill, happy or sad, calm or distressed. The light itself is your ability to be aware of these things, or self-awareness, if you prefer to think of it that way.

The light is *always emanating from you*. The ships will come and go. The shoreline will change. The tide will go in and out. The weather will at times be dark and stormy and at others bright and calm. Regardless of what the light is shining upon, it always comes from the same place—the lighthouse. As the lighthouse operator, you get to choose where the light shines and what gets illuminated. While the content of your life may change dramatically from time to time, maybe even from moment to moment, your awareness of it and your perspective of it always come from you and your choices. We have little control over the ships and the tides and the rocks on the shore, just as you had little control over whether or not you got bitten by a tick, a doctor recognized your symptoms, or you got adequate treatment.

As the lighthouse operator, you get to point the light wherever you choose and for whatever purpose you choose. The lighthouse, therefore, becomes a safe place to observe the events and content of your life, whether it's dark and stormy or there's a beautiful sunrise over a calm sea. Self-as-context seeks to accomplish the same thing—to enhance your ability to see the events and content of your life from a safe distance—objectively, flexibly, and with perspective. It's very difficult to see where the rocks are if you're in the ship during rough seas. But from the lighthouse, this is a much easier task. That's where you want to be, and that's where self-as-context seeks to take you.

Self-Stories

Let's face it, we all tell ourselves stories about who and what we are. We've done this from the moment we possessed the necessary language and cognitive abilities to do so. For the record, that's pretty young. It starts to happen very early in childhood. Those stories, whatever they may be, take your pick—*I'm too fat, no one likes me, I can't run fast, I'm not smart enough, I'm not worthwhile, I'm unlovable, everyone is better than I am*—have a tendency to stick with us. Even if we haven't been traumatized or victimized and lead relatively normal and healthy lives, we have those stories. Some are culturally infused, but most are the byproduct of life experiences. Getting chosen last for the team, being picked on, having a failure of some sort, receiving an unkind or unintentionally snide comment by a peer or even a complete stranger can sow the seeds of these self-stories.

It's at these times that our minds are working overtime. You might as well have Ernest Hemingway in your head weaving the intricate tales of just how awful a person you are, highlighting and reinforcing your every perceived fault and character flaw. We don't always think this way of course, but I would be hard-pressed to find anyone reading these words who can't, on some level, identify with this ride on which we all too frequently take ourselves.

When we're in this space and engaged in this process, we've got the beam of light focused intensely on the rocks and waves along the shoreline. In other words, we're letting the *content* of our lives define our sense of self. We have to remember that as the lighthouse operator we have the ability to shine the light wherever we want and whenever we need to. We have that sense of awareness and are capable of allowing everything in our lives to be as it is, but *we* get to decide how much attention gets paid to it because the light always emanates from *us*.

In short, we're doing ourselves a great disservice when we over-engage with these stories that are harmful or interfere with what we really want to do in our lives. Every time you limit yourself because you're living your life according to these stories—or what we might call acting out of self-as-*content* rather than *context*—you stop yourself from being flexible enough to do things that might be meaningful or beneficial to you. Maybe you don't ask for the raise because you think your boss doesn't like you or that you're not good enough for a raise. Maybe you don't even apply for your dream job or your dream college or ask out the person you like. Maybe, because as a kid you came to believe that your thoughts or opinions weren't of value, you don't confront the friend or family member or doctor who is telling you that your symptoms are all in your head when you *know* that you're really, really sick.

"I'm sick" is the self-story of people with Lyme or any other chronic illness. However, feeling unwell and having a self-story that says "I'm sick" are different things. "I don't feel well right now because of my Lyme symptoms" can lead to a healthy choice like resting or participating in an activity that is pleasurable but modified to your energy level. While having the self-story that says "I'm sick" can prevent you from doing things that are fulfilling. "I want to apply for this dream job, but I'm sick." (I won't be able to do a good job.) "I want to play with my kids, but I'm sick." (I will only disappoint them.) "I want to ask out my crush, but I'm sick." (Who could ever love me like this?) You can see how "I'm sick" becomes a placeholder for other deeper self-stories. How many times in your life have you limited yourself or made unhealthy decisions because of what these self-stories have told you?

It's important to note that no matter where you shine the light as the lighthouse operator, the hazards are still there. Just because you're not training the light on the rocky outcrop doesn't mean it's not present. It's not your goal to obliterate the rocky outcrop any more than it is to erase the stories of your life. Just as the rocks are part of the shoreline and seascape, those events are part of who you are. But they don't have to *define* who you are, or more importantly, what you do. The point of all this is simply that you get to decide when and where to pay attention to what you want to. You get to decide what stories matter and mean the most to you.

Noticing

How do we decide what stories to focus on? If our negative self-stories are so ingrained, so reflexive, then how do we even know where to shine the light? An aspect of self-as-context that can help increase this flexibility is the ever-present ACT technique of noticing. We saw it in defusion and acceptance and it is no different here. Notice what's happening at any given point in time in your life *and in your mind*. This is a big part of finding that space in which to flexibly experience your life in the present. Ask yourself:

- What's happening right now, in this moment?
- What story is my mind telling me right now?
- Does that story seem familiar?
- How does it go again?
- How does it typically end?
- Does this have to be my truth in this moment?

When you're able to notice and recognize these stories for what they are—just stories—it gives you the power and flexibility to do with them what you want. I often refer to this as "the greatest hits" to help my clients recognize that they're caught in the same old patterns of paying too much attention to a story they've told themselves too many times. Trust me, these stories are familiar to you. You've heard them over and over again. It's just like listening to an oldies radio station. There's a limited catalog of songs available, and you know all the words to all of the songs by heart. Your stories are the same thing. You know them inside and out and you've heard them a million times, but you don't have to sing along—you can change the station. This simple act of noticing what's happening rather than being consumed by the experience of what's happening can go a long way in helping you decide where you shine the spotlight.

Be Here Now, Not There Then

You may have noticed that the title of this chapter is not "You Are *Who* You Are" but "You Are *When* You Are." This is because

You Are When You Are: Self-As-Context

self-as-context is a present-moment process. "Be when you are" and take the events of your life as they come. Interpret them and their importance as the person you are now, not the person you once were. "Be when you are" and don't let past versions of yourself or negative self-stories interfere with the present moment.

I'll give you an example. I have a client who spent the better part of her adult life fairly depressed, relatively unassertive, and quite avoidant of all things that just might make her life better—seeking a different job, finishing her novel, pursuing a relationship, or just standing up for herself when the situation called for it. It was clear to me that what really mattered to her was her writing and getting a different job where she was treated with more respect and was doing something she enjoyed. As she was lamenting the state of her life, she spoke of how she could never get a job utilizing her writing talents because she didn't have a graduate degree in writing, and at this stage in her life (she was in her 50s), never would.

I asked why that was the case, and she was taken aback by the question. By this point, she had already done some very good work on improving her life and being more assertive, but she couldn't really answer the question in any meaningful way. "Well," she said, "I just don't see how I could do that." I gave her a homework assignment to research graduate programs in creative writing. Not long after that, she enrolled in one, earned her Master's in Fine Arts, finished her novel, and is now working hard to make a significant career move and publish her book.

Her issue was that she was assessing her situation based on her previous conceptualization of herself—not good enough, unassertive, and so forth—and not seeing her opportunity to better her situation by pursuing something that really mattered to her. Once she shook off that "self-as-content" perspective and shined the light on the things that mattered to her, the rest was history. Does that mean things weren't difficult for her at times?

Of course not, but she handled them with a self-as-context perspective that allowed her to be flexible enough to deal with those difficulties rather than avoid them.

This tendency to allow our past to dictate our present is all too common and is exactly why self-as-context is so important to embrace. It becomes especially critical if you've had a particularly traumatic event in your life or a past that has been fraught with difficulty and pain. Jennifer's case will highlight how self-as-context can increase psychological flexibility.

Case Example: Jennifer

Jennifer, a 54-year-old woman, came to me for treatment after a traumatic event in her life, where she was violently physically assaulted at her place of employment. For the past year or so, she had been experiencing all of the symptoms of post-traumatic stress—nightmares, avoidance of things associated with the traumatic event, intense depression and anxiety, pain, and a host of other difficulties and problems. She desperately wanted to get back to work because she loved her job, but could not conceive of being able to go back to the place where she was assaulted.

In the course of our work together, it came out that Jennifer had had a horribly abusive childhood and was victimized by family members, acquaintances, and strangers repeatedly from the time she was a little girl until she was an adult. Initially, our work started to bring up flashbacks—a re-experiencing of various incidents of abuse from her past. She initially found these to be very distressing (naturally) and engaged in all sorts of activities—distancing herself from others and being very guarded in her interactions—to avoid having to feel these emotions and difficult sensations. However, as she came to accept these events in her life and stopped avoiding her experience of them, she felt much stronger and more confident in her ability to deal with them when they came up.

When she went back to work, she noticed that she felt more attentive, more focused, and more rewarded by the work she was doing. She also felt less bothered by stimuli that had the potential to trigger memories of trauma experiences. She has been able to embrace her present experience of the moment-to-moment happenings of her life, and that has made a powerful difference.

Jennifer stopped living her life according to the same old self-story of being a victim. She doesn't even like to refer to herself that way anymore. As such, she is experiencing herself with awareness of the *context* of the present moment, not the *content* of her past. Her success is a perfect illustration of the self-as-context process in ACT.

Self-As-Context in Lyme and Chronic Illness

As you may have already gleaned, when it comes to Lyme and chronic illness, self-as-context processes can get a little bit tricky. The ACT model was designed primarily for people who have been suffering from psychological pain of all sorts. Psychological pain is often accompanied by traumatic life histories and negative self-stories. While ACT has been applied in the treatment of chronic pain (Scott, Hann, and McCracken, 2016) and other chronic illnesses like Multiple Sclerosis (Pakenham and Fleming, 2011), it may not be immediately evident to you how ACT in general and self-as-context in particular applies to you. You may not have a repository of self-stories that have held you back in your life or traumatic experiences that have crippled your ability to pursue what matters to you. What you have now is an illness that has turned your life upside down and ripped it inside out. So, given that, why shouldn't you hang on to your past, especially if it felt a whole lot better than your present?

These are all legitimate concerns, and they need to be addressed. You've read through how self-as-context applies to a variety of situations, so you understand the concept. Now it's time to apply it directly to your illness.

I Don't Have Any Negative Self-Stories

If you've managed to lead a relatively healthy, happy, and well-adjusted life up to now, I commend you for it. However, it's important to know that self-stories don't always have to reach "pathological" proportions to impact your life and be relevant to your past, present, and future. It's human nature to have insecurities, areas of weakness, and dark corners of ourselves that we're unsure of, afraid of, or maybe even unaware of. While I have no desire to crumble your life into a thousand pieces, if you can't identify these areas for yourself and how they've hampered you or kept you from experiencing your life in an unfettered and flexible way, you probably need to look a little harder.

Ask yourself, your friends, your family, and anyone else who knows you well what your blind spots are. Others often see our insecurities more readily than we do. What you find may surprise you. Even if it hasn't caused you all that much trouble in your life, it's still good to know. When your life gets turned upside down by a serious illness (or anything else), things you weren't aware of or that didn't have much impact on your life can become roadblocks. Maybe the roles you played in your life never caused you any trouble because you didn't have any conflict.

For example, say you never worried about having lots of friends because you always had lots of them. Maybe many of them have been seeing less and less of you because dealing with your illness has become hard for them and they can't handle being there for you. You might think *I'm not lovable* or *I'm always doing things for others without reciprocation*. Or maybe you never identified issues with being a provider for your family because you were always a good one. What happens when you can't work and your spouse now has to carry the load, plus pay huge medical expenses? You might think *I'm a burden* or *I'm a failure*.

My point here is that even if things had been going

swimmingly prior to you getting sick, there are probably some self-stories in there that maybe weren't a big deal but are now. Getting familiar with your "greatest hits"—and we all have them—is always a good idea and will help us to notice what's happening, be flexible, and root out those blind spots.

My Life Was Better Before I Got Sick

Of course your life was better when you were healthy. It's natural to want to maintain this point of view for as long as you can. Being present with painful experiences, physical or emotional, can be a difficult skill, but it exemplifies psychological flexibility. Your initial instinct is to try and be the person you were and stay in the life you lived versus the one you're living now. Things were better when you were well, so why not stay there? What could be the possible harm in this?

It simply isn't the reality. The fact of the matter is that you are ill and you are in pain. That's a hard truth to live with, but it's real. Aspects of your life may have been stripped away from you—your energy, your freedom, your health, your job, your role in the family, maybe even your home or your family itself. Under such dire and extreme circumstances, it's just as harmful to attempt only to live in your happy and comfortable self-stories from the past—*I used to be so healthy, I could do whatever I wanted*—than it is to let the dysfunctional ones keep you from living your life. Self-as-context is an in-the-moment process that requires you to be present in your current life experience. Anything else falls under the category of experiential avoidance, and this will do precious little to help you move forward and live as richly and vitally as you possibly can.

Is the content of your life more difficult than it was? Indeed. Are there more rocky outcrops on the shoreline you have to be aware of? Yes, of course there are. But from your perch in the lighthouse you can still direct that light to the things in your life that matter and are meaningful to you *in the present moment*.

"Be here now, not there then" applies to the good, the bad, and the ugly. However, in the midst of all of this, it's important to remember that the *content* of your life (your illness) *does not determine who you are*. It only plays a role in your life experience. When sitting on high in the lighthouse (self-as-context and perspective taking), *you* get to make the decisions about where to shine the light and guide the ships to where they're supposed to be.

The following story about a client I had with Lyme disease illustrates how self-as-context can be a powerful tool in being psychologically flexible. Rebecca was able to tap into this process, and it dramatically improved her coping skills and quality of life.

Case Example: Rebecca

Rebecca, a 45-year-old married woman, was a successful professional and by all measures had a pretty good life—nice house, a good job running her own business, family close by, lots of friends, and was pretty healthy, save the normal age-related issues that come with being 45 years old. All in all, life was pretty good for her and she had no major complaints.

Over a period of a few months, she began feeling very ill. She had all of the classic symptoms of Lyme disease—fatigue, joint pain, headaches, brain fog, cognitive difficulties, and neurological difficulties. Her Lyme test was negative, so she was not treated for Lyme for some time. As her condition worsened, it became clear that this was going to be a life-altering illness. She was no longer able to perform in her job and had to close her business. Her relationship with her husband became very strained, as he was ill-equipped to handle the level of care she required. Her family also began to pull away, becoming convinced that the root of her difficulties was "all in her head." They became angry with her and were sporadic in their support. Rebecca also began to feel her friends start to pull away as her illness became more and more prolonged. She began to get the feeling that her situation was too much for others to handle and that she was becoming too much of a burden to everyone.

This situation triggered a lot of Rebecca's self-stories, which included a deep-seated need to satisfy the people in her life often at the expense of her own well-being or what was good for her. This triggered profound feelings of anxiety, despair, and loneliness. These self-stories had been long present, but she was functioning well enough that she paid little attention to them even though they affected her deeply.

Over time she realized the people in her life, save a precious few, were not the people she had thought them to be. As soon as she was no longer able to be of service to them, but instead needed them to help her, they were either unwilling or incapable of doing so. As she got better with proper treatment, the pain of the loss of these relationships was dramatic. She got divorced, is more distant from her family, and lost a lot of friends that she considered to be close. Like many people who have their lives turned upside down by Lyme, she was grieving the loss of her old life.

In the midst of all of this, Rebecca recognized her self-story of having to over-serve others in order to get them to value her. She decided to shine her light on the people who were there for her. She found value in her true friendships and was able to let go of the "dead weight" of relationships that were burdensome to her.

Rebecca was only able to do this via engaging in the self-as-context process. If she had desperately hung on to her old life and her old self-stories, she would have essentially been beating her head against the wall to make her life work again. If she had hung on, she would have felt resentful of her family for not believing her while continuing to try and please, appease, and serve them. She would have taken the blame for her husband's choice to leave and might have ended up in another relationship with someone who was incapable of handling hardship. She would have lamented the loss of her business and lived in regret and shame. As much as Lyme tore her world apart, it also highlighted the good, the bad, and the ugly in her life that she wasn't seeing before, which was blocking her from a rich, meaningful, fulfilled life.

Defusion and Acceptance in Self-As-Context

As you will see in Chapter 9, no process related to psychological flexibility operates in a vacuum. They are all intimately connected. As such, for self-as-context in particular, defusion and acceptance can be very helpful in getting you to that place of perspective regarding the self. Many of the exercises we discussed in those chapters are applicable for self-as-context because, essentially, what you are doing is trying to defuse from unhelpful self-stories and engage in acceptance of who you are and the events and experiences you're facing in your life at this moment. Just as you have learned to defuse from uncomfortable or distressing thoughts regarding your illness, your relationships, your functionality, and your life, you can do the same thing in regard to unhelpful versions of your self-stories—past and present.

A major part of perspective taking in self-as-context is related to acceptance. There will be aspects of what you are experiencing right now that are distressing to you and may not be representative of who you want to be. However, while you're dealing with these very difficult circumstances in your life, you will have to accept things about yourself that may be hard. You might not be able to be as present for friends and family who are in need, or you might not be able to engage in some of the activities you would normally like to do (more on this in Chapters 7 and 8). Your only real choice here is to treat yourself with compassion and do the best you can. I'm betting that's how you would treat anyone in your life that you care about, so why treat yourself any differently?

Let's Watch a Game of Chess

There's one more metaphor I'd like to pass along, and it's an ACT classic that was originally presented in the seminal ACT book that started it all (Hayes et al, 1999). It's one of my favorites. I use it all the time with clients, and they connect well with it. Imagine a chess board with half of the pieces representing all of the good and positive thoughts about yourself and the other half of the pieces representing the negative thoughts and feelings about yourself. Generally, the idea in chess is to wipe out all of the pieces of the other color. In this case, we would want all of the pieces representing our good and positive thoughts and feelings to clear the board of all of those pieces representing our nasty uncomfortable thoughts and feelings, right? So, off we go on our quest to conquer the board and "win the game" so all we have left on the board are our "good thoughts and feelings."

The only problem is that in this particular game of chess there are endless pieces because this is how your mind works. Every time you wipe out a negative thought or a "bad" piece, another one just shows up to take its place. Also, every time you move a "good" piece (or have a positive thought) it tends to attract a "bad" piece (a negative thought). *Oh, I had a good day today and felt pretty well* is almost always followed by, *yeah, but just wait until tomorrow, it'll be a miserable day because I can't have two good days in a row*. In other words, the chess game becomes the never-ending battle of your mind. As hard as you might try to rid yourself of all of the "bad" pieces so you're completely comfortable with yourself, you just can't do it. It's a futile effort.

If you were in a place of real perspective taking, what part of the chess game should be represented by you? The "good" pieces? The "bad" pieces? If you guessed that you would actually want to be the chess board, you're learning! In ACT, the aim is to be in a place where you can observe all the happenings of the "battle" of your mind but not be too engaged in it. In the chess metaphor, this place of perspective taking is the board itself. From this place, the machinations of the mind are still occurring, but all you're doing is observing the process and not really engaging or being overwhelmed by it.

It's also worth noting that a functional chess board requires both colored squares to work. You can't play chess without having both black and white squares and pieces any more than you can't live your life without having both positive and negative thoughts and feelings. In this case, being the board is the equivalent of being the lighthouse operator because it allows you to experience your life and yourself from a place of perspective.

Conclusions

Before wrapping up this chapter, I'd like you to take a look at a quote about the self from the Buddha:

> The foolish man conceives the idea of "self." The wise man sees there is no ground on which to build the idea of "self"; thus, he has a right conception of the world and well concludes that all compounds amassed by sorrow will be dissolved again, but the truth will remain.

I believe the Buddha is essentially saying that the concept of the self is somewhat foolish and baseless. Ultimately, that process will be fraught with sorrow and distortions of truth. Only through recognizing this can we "dissolve the self" and be left with truth. What is the truth of which the Buddha speaks? Well, I'm not a Buddhist scholar and I don't want to get too philosophical here, but I think the truth of which he speaks is the enlightenment that comes with ultimate acceptance, unencumbered by our versions or stories of ourselves from the past. From a Buddhist perspective this would mean the dissolution of the self. From an ACT perspective, it simply means accepting one's self flexibly in the moment—self-as-context rather than self-as-content.

Lastly, in the quote from the beginning of the chapter, Ramana Maharshi talks about the relationship between the ego and the self.

> All bad qualities center round the ego. When the ego is gone, Realization results by itself. There are neither good nor bad qualities in the Self. The Self is free from all qualities. Qualities pertain to the mind only.

Essentially, the ego is analogous to the mind in ACT terminology. He is making the point that the true self is free of all qualities— it is pure. Those qualities we ascribe to the self are merely constructions of the ego or our minds. This quote is all about perspective taking and recognizing that what our mind tells us about our self is just that, our mind telling us something about ourselves. It's up to us whether or not we engage in it or act on it.

Lastly, being in a perspective-taking space requires us to be in contact with the present moment. This may mean a lot of different things to different people, but as we move into Chapter 6, I'll dig deeper into that process and help you to develop this skill. It can be difficult, at times excruciatingly so, but it's a skill and therefore can be developed. So read on, and enjoy the moment!

Chapter 6

Contact with the Present Moment

Realize deeply that the present moment is all you ever have. Make the Now the primary focus of your life.
Eckhart Tolle

Staying Rooted in the Moment

Contact with the present moment is the second of the "centered" processes essential to developing psychological flexibility. It is often associated with terms like mindfulness, being present, or more commonly sayings like "take time to stop and smell the roses" or "enjoy the simple things in life." While mindfulness is an essential part of contact with the present moment, the construct as a whole is bigger than any of these terms. The main idea here is that all that really exists is the present moment. The past has already happened and the future has yet to happen—as such they are only constructs of our mind. In other words, the past and future can only exist as a function of our current thought processes, which are happening right now in this present moment.

The problem is that as human beings we have a tendency to pay way too much attention to these thoughts about the past and the future and not nearly enough attention to what's happening in the present moment. As you have no doubt experienced, this inability to remain in contact with the present gets us into a lot of trouble and robs us of the moment-to-moment experiences of our lives. In fact, some would argue that it robs us of our lives altogether.

While contact with the present moment is an essential part of the ACT approach, the concept of mindfulness or being present wasn't created by the founders of ACT. Indeed, the philosophical, cultural, and spiritual approach of "being present" has been taught for thousands of years, predominantly from Eastern cultures and religions, such as Buddhism. However, this idea of being mindful and present as a way to experience one's life—both the pain and the joy of it—is the main differential component of the "third wave" of behavioral therapy. Many have written profoundly about this process and played major roles in the integration of mindfulness into Western approaches to medicine and psychotherapy, most notably Jon Kabat-Zinn. I encourage you to seek out and immerse yourself in some of the suggested readings regarding this topic. You will be deeply enriched by doing so.

It's a Skill, Not a Gift

Human beings have problem-solving machines for brains. That means we tend to be notoriously bad at staying present and not getting hung up on the past or worried about the future. Our minds are constantly hooking us into these places and pulling us out of the present moment. The good news is that you don't have to have any particular talent or innate ability to stay present. Mindfulness is really just a skill. And like any other skill, it can be learned with practice and patience.

When I say "practice" I don't mean shaving your head, taking a vow of silence, and meditating at a Zen Buddhist monastery for 40 years. As attractive as that option might seem at times, you don't have to do that in order to be mindful of the present. Real mindfulness can and should be practiced anywhere, anytime, while you're doing just about anything. It's called "active mindfulness." As long as there's a present moment at hand (and there always is), there's an opportunity to be mindful of that present moment, even if you're engaged in doing something other than just sitting quietly and meditating. You can be mindful while washing the dishes, taking a walk, or eating a meal. Whatever the moment brings, the idea is to be present with that, even if it's painful or difficult.

What I mean by "practice" is a consistent effort, not just in practicing the exercises in this book, but in being mindful in the day-to-day, moment-to-moment aspects of your life. Mindfulness can be tricky. It's one of those things where if you think about whether or not you're doing it, you're not doing it. Mindfulness is about being completely and totally focused on what's happening right now. The one thing I can promise you is that when you start *really* working at this, your life will get measurably better. I can also promise you that it's not easy. Your mind will try to pull you away from the present moment almost constantly. It's an exceedingly rare individual who can just be fully present all of the time. We have all kinds of demands in our lives and are getting externally and internally pulled in hundreds of different directions at any given point. This was true even before your Lyme diagnosis, so be gentle with yourself. Stop, breathe, and just take a moment to focus on that breath. And do it again when you catch yourself drifting.

Case Examples

It might help to revisit the case example from Chapter 5. Jennifer, who was terribly traumatized at her workplace, perfectly illustrated the process of self-as-context. But she did that with a lot of help from contact with the present moment.

The assault brought out all kinds of trauma from her past, but she was able to stay connected with the current version of herself and not remain stuck in the victim role of her past. As part of her trauma, she would frequently experience horrible flashbacks — an intense psychological re-experiencing of the abuse and trauma. When she struggled against these, it was very difficult for her to move through them. But when she opened up, observed, stayed grounded in the present, and let them pass, they were easier to bear. It was obviously still painful and difficult, but being focused on the *present rather than allowing herself to be pulled into her past made the road easier for her to travel.*

Similarly, most of my clients with Lyme and chronic illness also develop the ability to stay present. Intense illness has a way of forcing people to see that worrying about the future or lamenting the past is an added burden they simply don't have the energy for. When you're very sick, sometimes all you can do is focus on your moment-to-moment experience. Unfortunately, that's often about just getting through the drudgery of each day. But if you're more *intentional* about your contact with the present moment, it will allow you to connect with some meaningful aspects of your life and your experience even in the midst of a horrible illness.

It's Not Just You

I'll admit it, I struggle with this process of ACT—a lot. I've worked on it in varying ways in my life with frankly minimal success. What I've found is that in order for me to be really connected to my present, it has usually taken rather extreme circumstances—whether they be joyful or distressing—to get me there. That's not really what mindfulness is supposed to be about though. The idea is to be present for every moment of your life, not just the big ones, and this is where I falter. I still "struggle with the struggle." But what ACT has given me, and what I hope it can give you, is a sense that the struggle is not only okay but *expected*. Even if it feels constant, just keep bringing yourself back to the present and stay in it. I'm not always there and you won't be either, but treat yourself with some compassion, forgive, and just keep coming back. With that in mind, I'm going to talk about some of the simple things you can do to be more present in your life.

The Basics

Noticing

Probably the most fundamental aspect of mindfulness is the process of "noticing." I talked about observing your thoughts and your internal processes in Chapter 3, so you already have some experience with this. Being mindful and present is all about paying exquisite attention to, and noticing, the present moment. It may be your thoughts, physical sensations, emotions, the food you're eating, the flower you're smelling, or the conversation you're having—it doesn't matter. All that matters is that you're attending to it and nothing else.

You'll find that this is a shockingly difficult thing to do. We're just not wired this way. From an evolutionary perspective, our brains are designed to perceive threats. This is how we've survived as a species in a dangerous world. It's natural for our minds to attend to as many things as possible that might want to kill us, so becoming enveloped in noticing one particular thing is not a natural process for us. This is where noticing becomes even more important because as you're trying to be mindful it's critical that you notice when you get off track (which you most certainly will) and then gently bring yourself back to the moment. This will happen over and over and over again. Sometimes a mindfulness exercise will seem like nothing but a constant redirection from your bothersome mind. It's important to know, especially in the beginning, that this is perfectly normal. Don't judge yourself for it; just let it be what it is. As you keep redirecting and practicing, you'll eventually find yourself having to redirect a little less frequently and existing in the present moment a bit more often. Just don't think too much about being there!

Being Present versus Past or Future

Our minds have a pretty nasty habit of constantly dragging us back to the past—regrets, sorrows, should haves, if onlys, my life would be different if. It comes in all shapes and sizes and does us virtually no good whatsoever. I'm not saying you shouldn't learn from your past. Your past is important. It informs who you are and is part of the tapestry of yourself. But recognizing the impact of a moment of your past and learning from it is a whole lot different than missing your present because you're repeatedly turning over in your mind the events of your past and wishing for a different outcome. That's the perfect exercise in futility, yet we humans spend an awful lot of time existing in this space.

The future holds a similar allure to the mind. This is where the mind kicks into high gear and the control agenda emerges, trying to make sure that everything will happen just as you want it to, soothing you with a sense of control. Certainly there are things over which you have a fair degree of control. Chances are pretty good that if you wake up and go to work, you'll get paid. If you drive carefully, you won't get into an accident. If you take care of yourself, you won't get sick. But as you can already attest, these actions don't carry with them any sort of guarantee. We see this every day. Companies go out of business and people lose their jobs. People are injured or killed in car accidents through no fault of their own all too frequently. And you can do everything you possibly can to maintain your health, but you still got bitten by a tick and contracted Lyme or some other TBD—and your life changed because of it. So, attempts to control our future should be undertaken with the greatest of care and with our eyes wide open. Bad things can and do happen, and then we're left with a present that we didn't bargain for or expect.

The real question then is, how does focusing on a present moment that can be painful, heartbreaking, and at times, excruciating, help anything? My answer to this is rather simple— not *easy* but simple. To put it plainly, what choice do you have? Clearly, delving into the past will not change anything. You can't go back and not take the walk in the woods where you picked up the tick that bit you, or better treat an illness you had no idea you had. Engaging in that process only feeds your suffering. Similarly, over-exerting yourself to control your future can be just as futile. Plus, any changes you plan to make—seeing a more knowledgeable doctor, taking a different medication, or even just finishing this book—*are all in the future*. They do nothing to impact or affect your current circumstances, which is what you're feeling and experiencing *at this very moment* in your life. So, again, what choice do you have but to stay present?

Much like I discussed in Chapter 4, living in the present and allowing yourself to experience it fully without judgment or reservation but with self-compassion and openness can have a profound impact on your experience of your present moment and thus your life. I have seen this over and over again with my clients across all diagnoses and modes of suffering, including people with Lyme and chronic illness. There is something about leaning into your present-moment experience, choosing not to fight it, run away from it, or change it, but just embracing it fully for what it is by observing it, noticing it, and letting it be, that fundamentally transforms the quality of your experience of that present.

Note the term, fundamentally transforms the *quality* of the experience. Embracing and living in the present will not absolve you from emotional pain or difficulty, but it can change how you experience it in your life. This is the goal. Remember, ACT is not designed to help you feel *differently*, it is designed to help you *feel* differently. Noticing and embracing your present is a big step in this direction.

Embracing your present and being mindful doesn't mean we reject, ignore, or abandon the past or the future. Paying attention to these aspects of our lives is important for our survival, which is why we have this amazing skill. But over-attending to them can be simply disastrous. Your mind will try to drag you down that rabbit hole on a nearly continuous basis to no useful end.

Mindful attention to the present is our anecdote for this kind of suffering.

Using Anchors

You may have people in your life who seem to effortlessly accomplish this present mindedness. I am truly happy for these folks, but I am definitely not one of them. I struggle with this particular process every single day, sometimes every moment, of my life. I have a busy career and family life. As much as I love that about my life, it makes it easy for me to get pulled in a lot of different directions. I'm sure you feel the same way. Chronic illness holds a particular skill in making the mind busy with the past and the future and pulling us out of our present. That's why I like anchors.

I'll talk about our most important anchors, our values, in the next chapter, but I'm talking about something different here. What I mean by anchors is anything that mindfully grounds us in the present moment. Climbing a mountain can be an anchor for me, but it's not a realistic day-to-day anchor because I'm not doing that every day and I can't draw on it whenever I feel like I need it. Our sensory experience, however, is an ever-present anchor that is by definition experienced in the present moment. If you recall from the mindfulness exercise in Chapter 2, we used our senses to ground us in the present. We can access our sensory experiences—what we see, hear, smell, feel, taste—constantly. As such, our senses serve as excellent tools for grounding us in the present.

Anchors can also be hobbies, activities, values, or people—really anything that gets us focused on our present experience. Anchors are not, however, distractors that pull us away from feeling what we're feeling. Rather, they should be reminders about what true mindfulness is. If you have friends for whom being present seems relatively effortless, they could be anchors for you.

We need these anchors because if you listen to your mind too much, there's always plenty to worry about—as you know all too well. The point is to not hold on to those worries a moment longer than it serves you. These are the questions you need to ask yourself. How is holding on to this past or trying to control that future really serving you? Is it serving you at all or just paralyzing you, keeping you stuck? Just like with quicksand, the harder you try to pull yourself out of it, the deeper you get sucked in. But you get out of quicksand by spreading out, opening up, and allowing your body to come in contact with it as much as you possibly can. Allowing yourself as much contact with the present moment as you can, despite how scary it might be, is how you rise above the suffering of your experience.

Mindfulness and Lyme

My guess is that on some level you've experienced mindfulness before. Most people have, usually when they're deeply immersed in something they truly enjoy, whether that's competing in an athletic event they've trained for, taking a walk in the woods or on the beach, being with family, watching a favorite TV show, reading a great book, or eating a favorite food. All of these moments of mindfulness are wonderful when they happen and we should cherish and enjoy them as best as we can. The problem is that all of these things are enjoyable. It seems relatively easy to be mindful in those moments, doesn't it?

But what about being mindful when there's great pain, loss, hopelessness, or helplessness, such as what you may be experiencing as a result of your Lyme disease or chronic illness? Why would anyone want to pay exquisitely close attention to those moments, to embrace them fully as they are? Why wouldn't we just run away as quickly and as far as we possibly can? Distract ourselves from the pain in any way possible? Isn't that what we're supposed to do?

Well, you tell me. Have you tried doing that yet? Have you

tried running away? Distracting yourself? Living in your past? Tried to control every aspect of your future? Is that working? Do you feel any real relief from your pain? Are things better? Maybe for a moment or so, but nothing that lasts very long, right? This is my point—you've been doing everything else you can think of trying NOT to be present because the present is too painful. But what happens if you just allow yourself to experience your present, flexibly, and without judgment or reservation?

What happens if you spread yourself out across the quicksand instead of continually trying to pull yourself out of it? Does it *feel* any differently? If you choose to embrace your present, does it make the weight of your pain any lighter to carry with you? I don't know the answer to these questions for you, but I have seen this approach work and there's a mountain of scientific literature that supports the notion that this kind of flexibility can have a profound impact on your functioning and your experience of your life. Are you willing to try something different and find out the answers for yourself?

The Detective and the Documentarian

One of the ways you can move towards this kind of perspective is to move back and forth from being a detective with a magnifying glass and documentary filmmaker with a video camera. If you find yourself worrying, you're probably focusing on the past or future. This is a cue to get out your magnifying glass and turn your attention to what you see right now. Look at what is, not what could be or what was. If you find yourself frustrated by your pain and discomfort, put yourself behind the video camera and focus on the broader context of your life.

Chronic illness not only gives you a lot of time to think, but it also trains you to think about your illness…a lot. You've likely traveled a long road of doctoring and misdiagnoses and uncertainty that put your mind through its paces. So, you need to train yourself to stop running through imaginary scenes from the past or future. This is where the magnifying glass comes in.

Imagine Sherlock Holmes. He notices every detail in the moment, intently focused on his environment. When you catch yourself ruminating on your worries for the future and regrets of the past, float those thoughts away and channel your inner Sherlock Holmes. Pull out your magnifying glass and zero in on the present moment, whether it's listening to a friend, noticing how the air feels going into your lungs, or really tasting a sip of water. Just be in the moment. Put each detail under the magnifying glass.

This close-up perspective helps you to observe carefully and without judgment what you're experiencing. This can be a powerful way to allow yourself to experience whatever it is, as it is, openly and freely. It's great for positive moments and emotions, because being present in those moments is what the best of life is all about, isn't it?

Sometimes, though, getting too close can be a bit overwhelming or it just doesn't provide the right perspective. This is often the case when one is trying to be present with physical pain. Pain can be an overwhelming and dominant experience and focusing on it closely may not be helpful. At times like this, taking the director's seat can be more useful.

As the director of your documentary, you take a broader view. Sometimes you're sweeping the landscape taking in all of the colors of the fall leaves or tracking the crowded highway or panning the waiting room at the doctor's office. Sometimes you're on a familiar route, scouting a location and noticing an interesting feature you'd never really taken a hard look at. You can zoom in on a face or the texture of a fabric then pull back and capture a conversation, turning to one character then cutting to another. Like any good documentarian, point the camera at the action whenever possible. If you're with a friend, focus on what she's saying, the words she chooses, her vocal quality, and body language. And if you're alone taking some time to rest, notice your room, your body in repose, or a beam of light coming through the window.

You have to be careful here, because the documentarian view is not about trying to distance yourself from your pain—that would be akin to avoidance. It's really just about seeing your current experience of the moment in a broader context. Your pain is only part of the larger picture of your experience and your life. Yes, it is present and you do experience it, but you also experience love, joy, frustration, family, and any activity you're able to engage in. The video camera allows you to experience all of the present moments in your life, giving you a larger context.

You can also think of these two perspectives as the microscope and the satellite—zooming in on the minuscule then pulling back into the sky. Use any metaphor that works for you to imagine a close and broad view, then move between them as needed. For example, if your pain intrudes, give it a moment. Notice it. Breathe into it, then focus on your breath using the magnifying glass again. Catch yourself drifting and cycle through noticing the world around you at the moment from the point of the documentarian. Then take in the whole of your experience using your magnifying glass again to focus on your five senses in turn. You'll soon see that your experience encompasses so much more than your pain.

Being able to move back and forth between the focused and broad perspectives can be hugely powerful in helping you stay present, to experience whatever life is giving you *at* that moment *in* that moment, rather than trying to avoid or move away from it. We've already established that escape does not work in the long term, so trying new things is critical to developing the kind of flexibility that will help you to live an enriched and rewarding life no matter the circumstances.

Conclusions

Being present is a constant effort. It's something that ultimately you will experience as a series of failures until you realize that the only thing you ever need to do is recognize when you drift, forgive yourself, and redirect your attention to the moment. That second part is very important. So many of the people I work with get angry and frustrated when they find themselves drifting back into their old patterns. When they engage in that emotion it only takes them further away from the process. Notice and come back, notice and come back, and just keep going as best as you can.

Chapter 7

What Matters Most?

Life's up and downs provide windows of opportunity to determine your values and goals. Think of using all obstacles as stepping stones to build the life you want.
Marsha Sinetar

Leading a Values-Driven Life

For the better part of the last several chapters, I've been hammering home the point that it's not in our best interest to make decisions about our behaviors and our lives based on stories our minds tell us, emotional experiences we want to chase (or avoid), outdated versions of ourselves, or moments in which we've gotten stuck. Assuming you are on board with all of this to some degree, it begs a very important question. If we're not making decisions based on our thoughts, feelings, perspective of self, the past, or the future, then how do we know what to do in any given situation?

The answer to this is as clear as anything could ever be in the ACT model. It's something you've probably heard a thousand times before in a thousand different places from a thousand different people—your parents, teachers, friends, relatives, coaches, or even therapists. We need to make decisions, all of our decisions, based on our values. I recognize that this may be a loaded term for many people. It tends to conjure up notions of religion, morality, ethics, or laws—all of which *may* be related to your values but aren't necessarily. Values from an ACT perspective are yours and yours alone. Values work can be the best part of life, and I find it to be one of the most invigorating aspects of ACT. Once you identify what you live for, it's a touchstone that helps you see how life is full of experiences you can apply meaning to. From there, very little can stop you.

Values in ACT

It is not the intention of this chapter, this book, or ACT for that matter to define your values for you. While the word may carry with it a variety of connotations for you, some good, maybe some not so good, it's important that you understand exactly what I mean and how ACT defines and uses values to help you live a better life. From an academic perspective, Wilson and Dufrene (2010) describe values in the following way: "In ACT, values are freely chosen, verbally constructed consequences of ongoing, dynamic, evolving patterns of activity, which establish predominant reinforcers for that activity that are intrinsic in engagement in the valued behavioral pattern in itself." This is a mouthful, but let's take a closer look and see what they're really saying and what that means for you.

Values Are Freely Chosen

The fact that your values are freely chosen is fantastic news, because what it means is that this is one of the few areas in your life where you get to exert complete and total control. Assuming your values don't involve anything that advocates directly hurting others, such as abuse or assault, no ACT therapist or ACT book is going to tell you what you should or should not value. Where you may not be able to control your mind or your emotions, *you do get to control your values*. This is a primary difference between ACT and many other imposed value systems whether they're from religions, parents, or peers. While any of those groups may play important roles in how you decide what your values are, ultimately, YOU decide what they are—what matters to you, what's meaningful, and what direction you want your life to take.

The flip side to this is that freely choosing your values can be overwhelming. Many of us go through life so caught up in our pain or our attempts to avoid pain that we're completely disconnected from our own values. This contributes to a downward spiral in life and can lead to profound suffering. Ironically, when faced with the prospect of freely choosing one's values, people often freeze up, become paralyzed, or avoid the process altogether. Another reason for this is that our values are often intimately connected to our pain, which gets the experiential avoidance train running at full speed.

Values Are Action Based

As we've discussed, ACT is deeply rooted in behavioral principles, and values are no different in the ACT model. While we can certainly have feelings-based values, such as valuing the love of your family, ACT is far more focused on action-based values. In other words, *what do you **do** to move closer to what's vital, meaningful, and deeply important in your life?* Ultimately, ACT is about helping you develop psychological flexibility so you can lead a rich, vital, and meaningful life regardless of what pain you may be experiencing. In order for that to happen, you have to be engaged and action oriented. In short, no one gets what they really want out of life by having it drop into their lap. Meaningful lives come about as a result of action, and decisions about those actions need to be based on your values if you're to stay the course. Values serve as the guideposts for our decision-making processes. No matter how cloudy or murky our path may be, those guideposts will always bring us home.

Values Are Intrinsic

Engaging in values-based behavior is intrinsically rewarding. The value is in the behavior itself, not because it might bring some additional benefit. Sometimes an additional benefit comes anyway, and it's great when this happens, but the behavior is its own reward. This can be a difficult concept for people to grasp. For example, a lot of us work because we need to make money to pay the bills. But some of us work because we love the work we do. Sure, we get paid too, but the real reward is in the work itself, even if it's simply the value of doing something versus being unproductive. What really matters is the work, not so much the money.

There are countless examples of the intrinsic nature of values. For example, when I was deciding to write this book, I was advised by a colleague that it might not be a good idea for my academic career—I have a private psychology practice, and I'm a university professor. My colleague advised that I could move up in the academic ranks more easily if I concentrated on shorter-term achievements. What she said made sense, and this was helpful advice from a particular perspective, but the importance of writing this book surpassed my concern about the potential impact on my career. Would I love for this book to be a bestseller? Of course, but I'm not expecting that will happen, nor do I expect to get rich from writing this book. These would all be considered good extrinsic reasons for taking on such a task, but ultimately I'm writing this book because I want to help people who are suffering from Lyme disease and other chronic illnesses. I value sharing my expertise, caring for others, and supporting people in making their lives meaningful. If this book helps hundreds or thousands of people, I would be thrilled about that regardless of whether or not I made money or got promoted in the process.

I ask every client I see what it is that's truly important to them, what matters most in their lives, and I do it the very first time I meet them. Very few people tell me they want to be rich and powerful. Most tell me things like they want to be healthy, be a good parent, a good spouse, or make a positive mark on the world. This question helps direct where we're going and frame decisions in terms of their values. I refer them back to their answers often and help them further clarify their values throughout the therapy process.

However, it's not uncommon for me to get answers to that

question along the lines of what Russ Harris (2009) calls "Dead Man's Goals." I'll talk about the difference between goals and values in a moment, but essentially what he's saying here is that we should never set a goal or identify a value that a dead person could accomplish better than we could. When queried about what matters most to us, we will often make statements like "I just don't want to feel this way anymore" or "I want to stop doing" whatever behavior we've identified as problematic. These are all things dead people could do better than we can because they're phrased in a negative context—they describe inaction rather than action. The focus is on *not* doing something rather than moving towards something inherently meaningful. Values should always be phrased in the positive. Think of them as guidelines for behavior that you can always move *towards*. Dead people are really good at NOT feeling things and NOT doing things. We need to be the opposite.

This is particularly relevant if you're suffering from Lyme or another chronic illness. You're very likely to think about your life and your values in terms of what you don't want to be. You don't want to be sick. You don't want to be in pain. You don't want to be tired all the time. You don't want to have the symptoms you have. This is a natural response, but it has no place in determining your values because values have to be something you can move towards. Focusing on what you don't want to be will only contribute to you continuing to feel stuck. Framing your values as something you can move towards offers the potential for meaningful change.

Values Are Not Goals

Often when I ask what people value most in their lives they end up citing goals instead of values. They value graduating from college, having a job, or being a parent. Goals such as these are achievable and have an end point. Once they're reached, you set new ones and soldier forward. However, your goals are ideally supported by and grounded in your values.

Values are constant and are never really achieved. They are ever-present in our lives and are the criteria upon which we base all of our decisions. You're never done having values. For example, if I want to be a father, that's a goal, not a value. Once I have children, that goal is achieved and it no longer guides my decision-making process. However, if I want to be a *good father*, that's a value (a somewhat vague one, but a value nonetheless). Being a good father is something that I will never be done working towards (hopefully). Almost every decision I make in my life is infused with this value. If I think of the characteristics of being a good father—being present, expressing love and support, providing for my family, being a good husband to my wife, serving as a model for the kind of person I would want my children to marry—all of these things guide me in my decision-making processes, including how I interact with my children, what I do with my time, how I treat my wife, whether I volunteer at my daughters' schools, and so forth. I am never "done" being a good father.

Similarly, the values you identify can never be achieved or completed. If you think about the things that are important to you in the various domains of your life—work, family, health, leisure, spirituality—the values you connect to those things should be ever-present and serve as guideposts. They will always keep you on course.

Values Are Big Picture and Unifying

When asked to identify our values, we often respond with things we'd like to do or be. "I value my work" or "I value being a parent" might be some common answers to what you value. As I discussed earlier, values are action-oriented, but they should be identified with the quality of the action, not the action itself. While it's fine to value work or being a parent, it's more meaningful to identify the *quality of how* one works or is a parent.

For example, I value my work as a psychologist and a teacher, but there are qualities to that work that I identify as particularly valuable. Each provides an important service to others that hopefully enhances the quality and meaning of their lives. Both are intellectually stimulating and challenging and allow me to meet interesting people from whom I can learn (and teach) new things on a regular basis. It's these underlying qualities of my jobs that represent the real values of my work. It is also important to note that these things do not have to be specific to my work. I can learn new things, meet new people, and enhance the lives of others in a variety of ways and situations.

For anyone suffering from a chronic illness that may have robbed you of the ability to engage in the activities you love, identifying your values is absolutely critical. For example, it's pretty common for people who've contracted Lyme to have been "outdoorsy." It stands to reason that people who enjoy or value being outside would end up contracting Lyme since this is where ticks live. So, maybe you hiked, camped, or hunted a lot. After getting ill, your symptoms or treatment became barriers to engaging in these types of activities. You may have oppressive fatigue, sensitivity to light, and pain. Additionally, some antibiotics make exposure to sunlight flat out dangerous. People with Lyme often struggle with their inability to engage in these valued activities, and rightfully so.

However, if you dig deeper into the values "treasure chest" and look at the issue more globally, you might see that while the specific outdoor activity may have been enjoyable, it was enjoyable because it connected you to something you valued — maybe it was being close to nature, getting away from the hustle and bustle of day-to-day life, or doing an activity with someone you care about and being connected to that person in a specific way. As I mentioned, I love to climb mountains with my best friend from childhood. Probably 70 percent of the reason I do that activity is to bond with my friend. The activity is simply a vehicle for me to get to do what I really value—connect to another human being by sharing unique life experiences. At some point, we won't climb mountains anymore, whether it's because we're just no longer physically able or, as our wives would say, we've finally come to our senses. However, even though that activity won't be available to us, we can still connect with each other and make decisions that move us towards that value, not away from it. And that's what matters.

Typically, there comes a time in our lives when we can't do what we love as well as we used to. Athletes lose the physical ability to compete like they used to as they get older. Musicians can't play their instruments the same way they did when they were 25, or maybe they can't play at all anymore because of illness or injury. Lyme disease may have brought you to this point earlier than you wanted, but that time when we "can't" anymore *always* comes earlier than we want it to. So what do you do? When you realize that the love of the sport drives the athlete and the love of music drives the musician, you find other ways to engage with that love. Or maybe the athlete's value is in being competitive. If so, then the game may change but the satisfaction remains. The musician could simply enjoy being expressive or creative, which can be accomplished in so many fulfilling new ways. You coach, you teach, you write, you watch, you listen. You do anything you can to stay connected to what is ultimately the larger value. Vehicles that move us towards our values can change even if the value itself doesn't. You may not be able to drive the fancy sports car anymore, but you can still drive something—even an old clunker can get you where you need to be. The idea is to stay engaged with your values in any way you can.

Whatever activity Lyme or some other illness has taken from you, find out what it was about that activity that made it really matter to you. Why did you love being outdoors? Was it because you were connecting to nature? Seeing wildlife? Being with friends or loved ones? How else can you engage in that value in your life? If you loved your work that you can't do anymore, ask yourself *why* you loved your work. What was it about the job or the career that you really valued? Was it that you were accomplishing something? Did you enjoy being in charge? Helping others? Providing for your family? How else can you do that in a way that's possible for you now? The answers may not be perfect. Setting up a bird feeder outside your window may not be as thrilling as seeing wildlife in the woods, but that comparison is not a worthwhile thought to be engaging in. It's simply your mind trying to spoil your party and keep you from being in the moment and engaged with what matters most in your life.

Values can NEVER be taken away from you by anything or anyone. Lyme may have robbed you of the vehicle through which you used to engage with your values, but it cannot rob you of your values themselves—nothing can. No matter what has happened to you in your life, you can always make choices to engage in a values-driven life. It might not be pain free, as Victor Frankl knew all too well, but moving away from your values will only prolong and increase your suffering. As I said in Chapter 4, pain in service of living your life is just pain—pain in service of avoiding your life is suffering. Perhaps not surprisingly, when people are having difficulty identifying their values globally, guess where they often find them?

Want to Find Your Values? Look to Your Pain

Values and pain go hand in hand. If you're having difficulty identifying what your values are, what matters to you most, look to the pain you experience in your life. It's a fundamental principle of ACT that we can't lead a values-driven life without also experiencing pain. By necessity we often have to make choices that will move us towards what we value but will also cause us tremendous pain. Where we get into trouble is in our attempts to avoid experiencing any pain at all. That's how we end up off track and moving away from our values.

I had a client who went through a difficult divorce from an extremely emotionally abusive man. In the process, she lost custody of her young daughter and had to move out of state in order to make a living. After a years-long legal battle, she regained partial custody of her daughter but had to return to the state where her daughter and ex-husband resided. She had started to set down some roots where she moved, including a great job, a caring relationship with someone who made her feel safe, and a relatively good life. However, the new man in her life wasn't willing to move to continue the relationship, so she was essentially being forced to choose between the life she had built and returning to an environment that was in almost no way healthy for her, except that was where her daughter lived — affording her the opportunity to be more present and involved in her life again.

When we spoke about this horrible choice she had to make, everything about her resonated with a profound sense of despair and sadness. She had no idea what to do. Returning to her home state would end this safe relationship, reduce her earning power, and put her back in the proximity of her abusive ex-husband. Other than being with her daughter, there was nothing good about making this move. The pull of being in a happy relationship where she was well cared for, something that had never happened in her life before, was very strong, especially when coupled with the desire to avoid contact with an abusive ex-spouse.

To help her resolve her conflict, I asked her a very simple question. "What was the most painful thing you've ever experienced in your life?" Her answer was instantaneous and obvious. "Losing my daughter." At that moment, it all became clear to her. Despair turned to clarity and resolution. She made a values-based choice to be a present parent to her daughter even though it would most certainly involve a lot of pain and difficulty. In her pain, she was able to find and connect with her values. Thus, her decision became clear. It was not necessarily easy, but definitely clear.

Dealing with Values Conflicts

This case perfectly illustrates the fact that at times we have values that conflict. Even if we're well connected to what's important to us, sometimes we have to choose one value over another. We can value being in a loving relationship with a partner and being a loving and present parent, but sometimes life deals us a bum hand and we can't have both. This is an unfortunate reality of life, but it highlights two important aspects of values identification.

First, it's not a bad idea to have a rough sense of how your values are prioritized. You value things in various areas of your life, but some are undoubtedly more important than others. Having a sense of where those priorities are will help you when you're faced with values conflicts. My client valued both relationships and motherhood, but her fear clouded her priorities. Once she connected to her pain, this conflict was resolved relatively quickly. She was able to identify her value of being a good parent as more important than being in a safe relationship. Keeping your priorities in mind can help avoid confusion and indecision.

Second, values are to be used as guides, not rules. Sometimes, whether it's because of a values conflict or just human fallibility, we're not able to make decisions or engage in actions that move us towards our values. Beating ourselves up over this serves no purpose whatsoever. While we need to hold on to our values, we shouldn't crush them in our fists. We need to be compassionate and forgiving with ourselves when, on occasion, we don't make the "right" decision or fall down in our efforts to lead values-driven lives. Values are supposed to free us and guide us, not crush us under the weight of unrealistic internal expectations.

We do what we can when we can do it, recognize as best as we can when we aren't doing it, and gently redirect ourselves back on the values-driven path.

Values in Lyme and Chronic Illness

At this point, I think you have a general understanding of what I'm talking about regarding values, so let's turn to how values processes are important for those who are dealing with acute or chronic Lyme or another disease or disorder. It might be helpful to give you a case example of one of my clients with long-term, chronic Lyme disease for whom values clarification became very helpful in her life.

Case Example: Megan

Megan is a 56-year-old divorced woman who has been suffering from chronic Lyme for many years. While her Lyme treatment was helpful and she is far more functional than she was, she has lingering symptoms of fatigue, poor short-term memory, "brain fog," and other cognitive issues. She has a long history of depression and anxiety, which pre-existed but was exacerbated by her Lyme diagnosis.

Megan has two grown sons and also cared for her elderly mother, who was suffering from dementia and was recently placed in a nursing home. This was a very difficult decision for Megan and she had little emotional support from her siblings or children. She had been on disability and hadn't worked for quite some time, lived alone, and spent a good deal of her time in bed struggling with depression and fatigue. When she was able to get out of the house, it was usually to visit her mother at the nursing home.

In discussing values, I asked her what mattered to her the most and she responded accordingly—caring for her ailing mother, being connected with her kids, and taking care of her house. She was doing well with caring for her mom and kids but had been procrastinating on multiple projects around the house. She also enjoyed socializing but rarely went out and had no close friends.

When discussing in greater depth what she did when visiting her mother, she revealed that in addition to seeing her, she would visit with other residents of the facility, talking with them and engaging in other activities. She found this to be rewarding, so I suggested she seek out opportunities to volunteer doing this kind of work. With some encouragement, Megan was able to find such an opportunity at a similar facility in her area. She did so well that the facility offered her a part-time job.

The prospect of working again after so many years was overwhelming to Megan. She was worried about her cognitive issues, being able to make it through the day without her fatigue interfering, and the possibility of making mistakes that could harm residents. We discussed how much of the difficulty she had been experiencing was precisely because she was avoiding the opportunities available to her due to fear. Her bed was a safe place where no harm would come to her, but she was depressed from the lack of engagement with values-driven activities in her life. If she were to break the pattern, she had to accept that fear was part of the package and move towards what she valued anyway.

She took the job and ended up doing well. We developed simple strategies to help her stay organized and focused—making lists, using her smart phone to set reminders, being open and assertive about her limitations with her employer, being kind to herself, and suspending harsh self-judgment about her performance. She works enough to keep herself active and engaged, but not so much that she wears herself out. She's met people at her job that she likes and socializes with on a regular basis now and she's more on top of keeping her house organized.

Megan's case is an excellent illustration of someone who improved her life by engaging with her values. When Megan decided to accept the fact that she was going to be scared, she refused to make her life decisions based on that fear. Instead, she made decisions based on what she valued (helping others), and her life was immeasurably improved. It was not free of pain, fear, doubt, or even depression, but it was richer, more vital, and more meaningful.

Values in Lyme

As I mentioned earlier, nothing can strip you of your values—not Lyme or anything else. They are yours, they are freely chosen, they are present-focused, they need not be justified, and they are at the heart of every decision you make. While an illness or life event may make it harder, even impossible, for you to engage in your values in ways that are comfortable and familiar to you, there are always alternatives to engaging in values-driven activities. If you're clear about what it is you really value, then your decisions about what to do about any given situation at any given time should be clear to you as well.

In regard to Lyme and chronic illness, it's crucial to understand that while actions may become "smaller," values remain just as large and important. What I mean by this is that your activities may be severely restricted by your illness. You may be housebound or even confined to your bed with limited ability to engage in much activity at all, so the idea of doing volunteer work or just about anything else seems beyond the realm of possibility. I'm going to talk more about committed action in the next chapter, but it's worth pointing out here that if you're clear on what your values are, you can engage in them in some way. No matter how small that action might be—holding the hand of a loved one, resting, taking a deep breath, seeing an old friend for 10 minutes—it will almost always be better than the alternative, which usually consists of beating yourself up about how much you've lost or can no longer do. There's that pesky mind again, so be aware!

Values Exercises

Values work can be difficult. Not many people have lived their lives in a values-driven way or at least they haven't necessarily been aware of it or conceptualized it as such. Far too many people live their lives praying at the altar of emotional satisfaction or avoidance—which from an ACT perspective is pretty much the root of most suffering. So, figuring out what matters to you most can be more difficult than just asking yourself the question. You might get trapped into thinking that goals are values or actions are values. You might even construct a "dead man's" value. Thankfully, the ACT folks have done a lot of work creating exercises that will help you to construct your value system—and it *is* a matter of construction. Your values are all yours. You have complete and total control over them, so relish that because it doesn't happen often!

As with most of the ACT exercises in this book, these techniques are presented in other works as well. The ones listed below are taken or adapted from a list created by Russ Harris (2009) who has done amazing work in making ACT accessible to everyone. Again I encourage you to avail yourself of these additional resources. Mine is but one voice, and you will be far better served by seeking out the voices of others as well. The exercises below are designed to help you construct your values. I don't expect that all of these will resonate with you (nor should they), but I do suspect that some of them will. You won't know which ones will do the trick for you until you try them.

Speeches

Picture some event that's being given in your honor—a birthday party, anniversary, retirement, graduation, or even your funeral if you're comfortable going that far. At events like this, people give speeches about the guest of honor (you) that reflect on how their lives have been affected by you, what you stand for, what you meant to them, etc. Assuming you lived your life as the person you want to be, what do you imagine these people saying about you in their speeches? How kind and compassionate you were? How helpful you were in their times of need? Your honesty and integrity? Energy and enthusiasm for life? Willingness to try new things? Your loyalty? These are just examples, of course. It's your family and friends speaking about you, your life, and YOUR values. What would you hear? I sometimes refer to this as the "It's a Wonderful Life" method of constructing your values. I don't think many of us strive to be Old Man Potter, but that movie made it pretty obvious what really mattered to George Bailey, even if he didn't know it at the time.

Mind-Reading Machine

Think of someone in your life who's very important to you — a spouse, best friend, parent, or child. Now imagine that you could place a mind-reading machine on their head that would tell you everything they're thinking. As you do this, you discover that they're thinking about you. What do you want to hear them say to themselves about you? In a similar way to the previous exercise, focus on the important stuff, not whether or not they like your new haircut. What do they think about the kind of person you are, what you mean to them, what you stand for? If you lived your life in an ideal way, what would you want to hear them thinking?

Life and Death

Imagine that you only have 24 hours to live but can't share that information with anyone. What would you do? Where would you go? Who would you see? Being ill puts this exercise in an entirely different light because it forces you to consider your own mortality in ways that you may not have done when you were healthy. Rather than focus on the fear, use it to discover what really matters to you. Illness can help you focus your values in very sharp and distinct ways if you let it.

Wealth

Just about everyone has imagined what they would do if they hit the lottery or inherited a fortune, but this can easily be turned into a values exercise. When practical or financial barriers are removed and you're free to do whatever you want, what would it be? With whom would you share your newfound wealth, both in terms of the money and the time and experiences you'd have? Thinking about this will help you construct both what and who is meaningful in your life.

Exploring Your Pain

I touched on this earlier in the example of my client whose most painful moment helped her realize what she really valued. If you think of pain as your ally, it can tell you a lot about what you care about and who matters to you the most. It can also teach you to grow, learn new skills, and become stronger. Just as no athletes excel in their sports without the pain of training, you can't grow in life without experiencing pain and loss. It shapes and forms us in ways that we're often resistant to, but are vitally important. Your fears, anxieties, worries, and pain also tell you what you care about.

Character Strengths

I ask this question of every client I see in the very first session, and it's often the hardest one for them to answer. They will spend an hour and a half telling me about their pain and all of the things that are wrong with their lives (and themselves), but I'm often met with stunned silence and bewilderment when I ask, "What are your best qualities? What do you like most about yourself?" Of course your pain is important, but so are your strengths. Know them, embrace them, and identify other things about you that you want to develop and grow.

Magic Wand

There are two layers to this one, both designed to get away from the external factors that interfere with the choices we make. First, imagine I wave a magic wand and all of a sudden everything you do is met with full approval from everyone in the world. No matter what, you would be universally liked and respected, whether you were a philanthropist or an axe murderer. What would you do with your life, and how would you treat others?

Second, imagine that I wave the magic wand and all painful thoughts, feelings, and memories don't affect you anymore. You essentially get to lead a pain-free life. What would you do? How would your life change? What would you do more of? Less of?

What Matters

What matters to you is the theme of this chapter. So, simply ask yourself the question—what matters? For some people the answer to this question is instantaneous and obvious. Other people need to probe a bit. What do you really like and enjoy? What do you want to stand for? What kind of person do you want to be? Is there anything in your life that excites you or energizes you?

The Sweet Spot

Take a moment to settle yourself—ideally you would do a brief mindfulness exercise—and then as vividly as possible, recall a moment in your life that was sweet, touching, or prompted some sort of positive emotional response. What was it about this response that was so meaningful? How is that connected to your values and what's important to you?

Disapproval

Just as it is important to identify what is meaningful to us, we can also learn from things that we don't like or disapprove of, especially in the actions of others. Perhaps you don't tolerate rudeness, dishonesty, or laziness. Knowing what you don't appreciate and where that comes from can lead to important insights into what really matters to you, how you want to conduct your life, and the choices you make.

Missing Out

This brings back our old friend experiential avoidance. Think about whether or not there is anything in your life that you're holding back from and not engaging in because of a lack of willingness on your part. Are there things in your life you're not doing that you would like to do simply because you're avoiding some painful aspect of that activity? Do you value being healthy but aren't exercising like you'd like to because it can be difficult? Is there something you'd like to do but are avoiding it because you're worried about how Lyme interferes with it? Remember Megan and how long she missed out on doing something meaningful because she was afraid she wouldn't be able to do it? What are you missing out on?

Childhood Dreams

Think back to your childhood dreams. What kind of life did you want for yourself? How close are you to hitting that mark? Are the same things important to you now that were important to you then? If not, how have they changed? How is your life different from what you imagined it would be? What significant choices have you made that put you on your path? Are you stuck holding on to a previous version of yourself? Or is that previous version of yourself helping to guide you through difficult times?

Likes

Quite simply, just ask yourself what you like to do. Then ask yourself what it is about doing that thing that you really like. I discussed this earlier in the chapter as well. Identifying the underlying aspects of what you really like can help to construct your values and guide your choices.

Role Models
Think of someone you admire and look up to. It could be someone close to you, but it doesn't have to be someone you know. It could be an historical figure, leader, or innovator. Think about the characteristics and qualities they possess that you admire the most. What are their strengths? What do you admire about them? How are you like them? What aspects of yourself would you like to possess to become more like them?

Forms and Worksheets
In addition to the visualizations and mental exercises described above, there are many values worksheets that will help you explore your values in the different domains of your life—family, relationships, work, education, leisure, health, personal growth, and spirituality—that are available either in other ACT texts or online. A simple internet search will turn up many that might be useful to you. Some of the websites that contain versions of these forms are listed in the resources section in the back of the book. I encourage you to use these resources in addition to what's described here. While engaging in mental exercises can be helpful, writing things down has a unique effect in solidifying the information and connecting more concretely to it. You could do any of the exercises above in written form as well.

Conclusions

While each of the core processes in ACT is essential, I believe that values play an important part in holding the model together. ACT is unique in this regard compared to other modes of psychotherapy. I view it as a major strength of the model and an essential element of developing psychological flexibility.

While you might be swimming in the sea of defusion and acceptance and working hard to stay in the moment, values are the grounding force that brings it all together and gives your life meaning. We can defuse more easily from unhelpful thoughts if that leads us towards our values, and we can more willingly accept painful emotions and events in our lives if they're in service of what we hold dear. Doing all of that requires that we stay present. If we leave the moment, chances are we're off track. If, however, we keep bringing ourselves back, we position ourselves to make real and lasting change. Not surprisingly, since ACT is rooted in a behavioral approach to change, to really make that leap requires actually *doing* things differently. This brings us to our final process of psychological flexibility — Committed Action.

Chapter 8

Doing Is Living: Committed Action

Any action is often better than no action, especially if you have been stuck in an unhappy situation for a long time. If it is a mistake, at least you learn something, in which case it's no longer a mistake. If you remain stuck, you learn nothing.
Eckhart Tolle

It's Called ACT for a Reason

Committed Action is the last of the six core processes of ACT, and this is pretty much where the rubber meets the road. You've increased your Openness using Acceptance and Defusion. You've become Centered from Self-As-Context and Contact with the Present Moment. And you're halfway to being Engaged with your Values firmly in place. Now you get to make values-based choices and take values-based actions where every present moment has a higher purpose and each choice develops a pattern that supports what matters to you. Essentially, this is where you get to put it all together by engaging with behaviors that will make your life better.

As defined by Hayes et al (2012, p. 328), "committed action is a values-based action that occurs at a particular moment in time and that is deliberately linked to creating a pattern of action that serves the value." That's a relatively short and simple definition, but it's packed full of important concepts, not just for committed action but for the ACT approach overall. Notice that committed action is intimately and explicitly tied to values. I'll talk more about this later, but it warrants mentioning here that the purpose of ACT is to move you towards something that's important to *you*, that *you* value, that *you* find meaningful. Values without action are useless, and actions without values are directionless at best, destructive at worst.

As you may recall, at its core ACT is a behavioral approach. What this means is that *doing* is critically important. Without doing, nothing happens. You remain stuck in your life, unable to move forward and often repeating the same old patterns. If you want a different outcome, you can't keep doing nothing or doing the same thing over and over that isn't working. This is what the "C" in ACT is all about, *commitment* to an action that works for you—and by "works for you" we mean moves you towards what you value. This is such an important process that the very acronym of the approach reinforces the necessity of it.

You Own It, so Own Up to It

For many people, the idea of action is simply overwhelming, daunting, or just plain scary. We get cold feet or get caught up in the "what ifs," responding or non-responding based on fear and whatever line of nonsense our minds decide to feed us at any given point in time. *What if I can't do it? What if I fail? What if I make things worse? What's the point? It won't work anyway.* We've all heard these statements or some variation of them ramble through our minds at different times in our lives. And I would guess that we've all too often let these words dictate our actions. That doesn't have to be your reality.

The scary part of committed action is the flip side of this process. I've spent a good bit of time convincing you that trying to control the thoughts that rattle around in your mind or the feelings that run through your body is largely a useless exercise. I've talked about the dangers of the control strategy and emphasized the need to allow yourself to feel and think what you are feeling and thinking in the moment without judgment and as flexibly as possible. That presents challenges, of course. But committed action, much like your values, is where you get to call the shots. While you may not have much, if any, control over your own thoughts or feelings, you have essentially total control over your own behavior. In the same way that you get to choose your values, you get to choose your actions and behaviors. This, of course, doesn't mean that we get to do whatever we want whenever we want. I think we can all agree that there are situations where we simply cannot act in the way we want, for example, when we are too ill to do so. However, that doesn't mean that you can't act in *some* way that moves you closer to what you value. This is a powerful distinction that gives us a much broader range of options than we may have expected or been aware of—and that broader range can make all the difference in the quality of your life.

An important thing to remember in ACT (and in your life) is that you bear the responsibility for both your action and your inaction. Both are based on decisions. (Yes, you can decide *not* to make a decision.) What we don't do defines us as much as what we do. However, it's through doing that we live and through waiting that we wither. If you're waiting and not doing, it's within your control to change. Take a moment to recognize the ways in which you're waiting, stalling, and withering. What are you waiting to do? When you think about what you want but don't have, what do you tell yourself? Simply pay attention to what you're thinking and, without judgment, identify your excuses, justifications, or perfectly reasonable arguments as "inaction." Now that you see where you're stuck, you can make the necessary changes to move your life in a meaningful direction. Again, you may not be able to do *exactly* what you want, but if you can do *something* that moves you in a valued direction (and you almost always can), this is better than doing nothing.

The Power and Pitfalls of Choice

If you own it and you have to own up to it, then that means you have a sense of agency or choice regarding your actions. Ultimately, this is a good thing, but we often experience choice as a burden, weighed down by the fear of making "bad" or "wrong" choices versus "good" or "right" choices. ACT doesn't focus on the moralistic aspect of choice. Instead it focuses simply on making one aware that choice exists. If you can let go of the weight of good/bad/right/wrong in regard to choice, it frees you up to simply think of a choice as useful or not.

To know if a choice is useful, you can evaluate it by whether or not it supports your values. Simply put, at any given moment, any decision or choice you're making is either bringing you closer to your values or moving you farther away from them. When viewed this way, choice is a powerful tool, an ally, in your quest for leading a values-driven life full of meaning and enrichment.

The Myth of Motivation

This is going to sound weird, but I don't think there's anything that facilitates procrastination and lack of action more than motivation, or more specifically, our concept of what motivation should be and how it should manifest itself in our lives. We are culturally inundated with what I consider to be dysfunctional messages about motivation. We see news pieces or read articles about exceptional individuals who do exceptional things— athletes, business people, astronauts—and the hidden message is that you have to be super-motivated to do anything important or useful. If you're not, well then you'd better get motivated or your life won't amount to anything.

The reality is that yes, these people are motivated, but people mistake motivation for ease. *Sure, that person can run 26.2 miles because they're motivated to do it, so it's easy for them, but I'm just not motivated to be fit, lose weight, eat right, etc.* If we actually sat down and spoke with anyone who has accomplished something difficult—or anything at all really—they will tell you that more often than not, they weren't feeling particularly motivated when they were doing their early morning workouts, or running their company, or studying hard to pass qualifying exams, or getting lunches made for the kids before they left for school. Ask anyone who's lost a significant amount of weight and they'll almost always tell you that it was a moment-to-moment struggle, that decisions had to be made every minute of every day, and that they did not always *feel* motivated—in fact most of the time, especially in the beginning, they probably wanted to give up.

They will also tell you that despite all of that chatter (thank you, mind!), they decided to act in a way that moved them towards their value—whether it was health, knowledge, serving their community, country, or family. Often, the motivation, feeling good about doing what was "right" for them, did not come until AFTER the action. In other words, the myth of motivation is that it has to come before the behavior. More often than not, the *behavior* actually facilitates motivation. You see, what people mean when they say "I'm just not motivated" is that whatever behavior they really want to act on is not going to be easy. "I'm not motivated" is really "this is too hard, if I were motivated it would be easier."

This leads to a subversive trap. You feel like you can't do anything until you're motivated, but as we know, motivation is elusive. Your brain is smart and over-protective of you—it will direct your body to rest and conserve energy as much as possible. It steers you away from hard work that it doesn't deem necessary for immediate survival. The mind convinces you that action is too hard and it's best to just stay put. Sure, once in a while you feel the urge to take action, but if we only took action when we felt like it, we would all be perpetually stuck.

The escape from the elusive trap of the motivation myth is to stop paying attention to how motivated you are, connect your actions with your values, and act accordingly. Notice that second part—*connect your actions with your values*. This is the other piece of the puzzle that most people miss. We tend to act or not act based on how we feel rather than on what's really important to us. If you remember that everything you do is enriching your life in some way, you can quiet the mind chatter—be it fear, entropy, or self-destructive self-talk—that sabotages action. We forget that we're doing something because it's actually important to us on a deeply personal and meaningful level. Thoughts and emotions can be loud, annoying, and interfering, but it's up to you if they determine your actions or not. Motivation actually has precious little to do with that process.

Ironically, what people will often tell you is that at some point if you keep acting in your valued direction despite how motivated you may or may not be, the motivation eventually comes. Anyone who has exercised on a regular basis knows that the first couple of months are just brutal. But after a while, you start to look forward to your workouts, and it gets a little bit easier. Not all of the time, but more so than it was before. So, action actually facilitates motivation (not the other way around). It's a cruel irony. But once you open up to action regardless of motivation, it's a powerful skill and will lead to an enriched life. John is a perfect example of how to break through the myth of motivation.

Case Example: John

John, a 34-year-old man, developed Lyme from an unknown tick bite, possibly years before his actual diagnosis. He had a preexisting complicated history of mental illness and was on multiple medications. All of this made his diagnosis difficult, as everyone attributed his symptoms of fogginess and paralyzing fatigue to his mental illness or side effects from the medications he was taking. He was holding down a full-time job and was in a graduate program when he was diagnosed. As he started to get treatment, the reaction to his IV antibiotics exacerbated his symptoms, making him feel worse. He endured extensive antibiotic treatment (both IV and oral) for almost 2 years. His fatigue was absolutely staggering, and his level of motivation for even the easiest of things was virtually non-existent. Despite this, he continued to work full time, commute an hour each way twice a week to his graduate program, and do well in his studies. John made his decisions to act based not on how he felt—if that had been the case, he never would have kept his job or stayed in school—but on what he valued and what he knew was important. He demonstrated that you can accomplish things you may not have thought possible whether you feel motivated in the moment or not.

I Promise, It Will Hurt (but not all of the time)

A big reason people stay stuck and lost in a sea of inaction is simply avoidance of pain. Whether it's emotional or physical pain, we try the best we can to avoid it. It's our natural inclination, and no one should be judged for it (by others or ourselves). But the fundamental reality is that inaction for the purpose of avoiding pain is not an effective way to live our lives. As I mentioned earlier, our values and our pain lie very closely to one another. Often, you simply can't get to one without going through the other. This is why we must remain open to experiencing pain or discomfort *in service of that which we value*. This means that engaging in committed action will often lead to discomfort—emotional, physical, spiritual, psychological, or all of the above.

If we allow our fear of that pain to dictate our actions, we are essentially adrift, which in and of itself is painful. Pain that is born of avoidance quickly turns to suffering. Once you decide to move, to take action towards a valued direction, *that* pain or discomfort has a purpose—and this can make all the difference. Sure, occasionally our values-based actions are flat-out easy, even fun. When this happens, ride that wave! Open yourself up to it, enjoy it, revel in it, and remember it. When you're having difficulty, you can remind yourself that acting in accordance with your values is not always a painful process.

Goal-Directed Action versus Value-Directed Action

In the context of committed action, it's critical to understand the distinction between goals and values. While goals are important, if all of our actions are undertaken merely as a means to achieve a goal, we're setting ourselves up for a fairly miserable existence. Goals, by their very nature, are future-oriented. You have a goal to feel well, to exercise more, to be more financially stable, or cure your illness. Even if you're acting in accordance with achieving these goals—following your doctor's recommendations, walking every day, saving money—the default set-up is that you won't be happy until you've achieved said goal. In other words, because goals are future-based, you can't be satisfied until some undetermined point in time. As such, you're robbing yourself of your ability to feel satisfied or happy in the present.

Needless to say, this is antithetical to the ACT approach. ACT is all about embracing the present moment flexibly and fluidly, free of judgment or reproach. With values-directed action, you can experience the satisfaction of engaging with your values on a moment-to-moment basis. Every time you make a deposit in your savings account, it feels good because you're engaging in values-directed, committed action. You get to enjoy every step of the process, not just the instance when you've met your savings goal. Every moment you're exercising or moving your body feels good because it's supporting your value of health. Every time you follow through on a medical treatment plan, you experience the value of that action, not just when you're "cured."

Of course, I am not saying that goals aren't important or that we shouldn't make them. I am saying that your goals need to be in line with and serve your overall values in all areas of your life. I'm also saying that connecting actions to goals rather than values is inconsistent with your ACT-driven commitment to staying present because goals are by their nature future-oriented. Most people do not consider these distinctions. But once you do, the shift in your approach can have a powerful impact on your day-to-day, even moment-to-moment existence.

Barriers

The barriers to engaging in committed action in a valued direction are many, but the good news is that you've read them all in this book already. If you've been paying attention, none of this will shock you, and you will already have a sense of how to overcome them and get moving. The big three barriers are the *stories we tell ourselves*, the *feelings we try to avoid*, and a *lack of connection to our values*.

We have all engaged in that mental back-and-forth when we argue with ourselves over what we're going to do—what we eat, whether or not we exercise, do our work, or mindlessly watch TV—these are all variations of the same theme. If we really listen to what our mind is telling us in these moments, we'd see the set-up. *It's too hard. I don't want to do that right now. Wouldn't it be more fun if,* and my personal favorite, *I can do that later.* Or maybe it's that you're not good enough, you might fail, you might embarrass yourself, or others might get mad at you. You know the drill. These are all versions of the stories we tell ourselves, and all too often it's the "same old story." If you take the time to notice this process, recognize the story, and then defuse from it (remember that?), you increase your chances of doing whatever value-directed action it is that you really hope or need to be doing. In other words, like I mentioned before, your inherently lazy mind will try to trick you into non-action. If you can notice this and defuse from it, your life will get better.

Similarly, because value-directed action will often carry with it some sense of discomfort, if not outright pain, you have to embrace difficulties. If we choose to avoid them, the easiest way to do that is simply to take no action. But we've covered that ground already, and we know that doesn't lead to much good for us. So, not surprisingly, acceptance becomes an important part of the committed-action process for us. If we're not willing to openly receive pain and discomfort in service of our value-directed actions, then we will not grow or enhance our lives.

Lastly, if for some reason our actions are not tied directly to our values, it is unlikely we will be successful. This can happen for any number of reasons. We may not have clearly delineated our values in the first place, we may be more goal-focused, or our values may have changed over time. If you are paying attention to these processes and making sure that you're in touch with your values, it will facilitate committed action.

I'll throw in a bonus barrier here, and that's simply what I refer to as "going too big." Successful actions usually come in small steps. It's a rare occasion when we bite off more than we can chew and find that meal nourishing—more often we end up choking on it. It's a common strategy in goal setting to make smaller, realistic, achievable goals. This is a wise strategy in taking committed action as well. When working with clients, once we identify a value, I will often ask them what kind of actions they can take to move towards that value. They almost always come up with some grand idea or plan that's far too overwhelming to them and ends up shutting them down. This is where we learn that even the smallest steps towards value-directed action can be powerful. At the very least, we can be assured that it's more likely to lead to a better outcome than doing nothing.

Willingness

Engaging in committed action requires openness and willingness to experience whatever may come. The most common reasons for people not engaging in committed action are what I've already listed—fear, avoidance, doubt, etc. If one doesn't adopt a certain amount of willingness to experience those consequences along with the action, then paralysis continues. We have to disabuse ourselves of the notion that everything has to be okay before we act. Life is too messy to be able to accurately predict the outcomes of what we do every single time, so willingly embracing some level of doubt and discomfort is a prerequisite for action. I'm certainly not saying we should act carelessly, but I've seen too many people spend too much time and effort trying to control every aspect of every outcome of every action to the point where they never actually get a chance to engage in any action at all.

Willingness goes somewhat hand in hand with acceptance, so the exercises we did in Chapter 4 will help you to embrace the discomfort and move forward in whatever actions you deem *useful* to take. Naturally, by *useful* I simply mean moving you towards your values.

Committed Action and Chronic Illness

As is often the case, things get a bit tricky when we apply these principles to situations surrounding chronic illness. More often than not, you might find yourself desperately motivated to do something, but you simply can't. You may be physically unable, utterly exhausted, or experiencing severe side effects from treatment. Lyme in particular can cause such a wide range of symptoms that affect so many different areas of your functioning that the very idea of doing anything can not only seem overwhelming, but may actually be out of your reach or beyond your current limitations. This might seem like it flips the script somewhat, but the answers remain the same.

In the context of Lyme or other chronic illnesses, there is no action too small, and sometimes inaction is the best action of all. The bottom line is that as long as you're connected with your values and acting in a way that moves you towards them, you're doing okay. For example, you may desperately want to play in the yard or at the playground with your kids or grandkids, but you simply aren't able to do it. It either hurts too much, you're too exhausted, or you know that level of activity will have an effect on you that would be harmful to your well-being. As such, the playground is off the table, but this is where your choice point lies.

What is the value associated with this activity? You most likely want to spend time with your kids or grandkids to be a good parent or grandparent, to foster some kind of caring, loving, relationship with them. If you invest all of your energy in lamenting the fact that you can't do that one activity with them, then bring on the depression, anxiety, shame, regret, fear of failure, and the whole cavalcade of unhelpful emotional consequences. However, if you stay connected to the value (fostering relationships) and not the action (goal) then you have a lot more flexibility here. Goal-oriented thinking would be "I want to play with my kids or grandkids at the playground." This is a worthy goal, of course, but what are you supposed to do in the meantime? Wait until that happens before you do anything with them?

If, however, you're connected with the value "I want to have a close relationship with my kids," the playground is but one activity in the realm of possibilities for making that happen. There will undoubtedly be many others outside of your reach, but which ones are within your reach? Can you read with them? Watch their favorite TV shows? Talk with them about their day, just listen to them, or tell them about you and your life experiences? The activities would vary depending on the age, of course, but there are many ways to relate with family members. The inflexibility comes from a rigid focus on the action rather than a global and flexible view of the value.

The bottom line is that illness will undoubtedly reduce the repertoire of available actions you can commit to in service of your values. Some of what has been taken from you is without question painful—probably excruciatingly so. However, you can always make choices that move you towards, not away from, your values. If you're consistent in this approach, your life will have more meaning than it otherwise would. Will it be what you want it to be 100 percent? Will you have the life you feel like you deserve, that you envisioned for yourself, that you counted on?

Maybe not. But I promise you, focusing on what you lost (rather than what you have) will not lead to any kind of meaningful existence for you or those you love. In whatever way you can, no matter how small, *engage, engage, engage.*

Megan Revisited

Committed action is an important process that I work on with all of my clients, especially my clients who have Lyme disease. Because Lyme can leave you feeling so robbed of the ability to do anything in your life, it's important to connect with what you can do. Megan, from Chapter 7, is an excellent example of how committed action can lead to improvements in your life despite how Lyme may have ravaged it.

If you remember, Megan came to me after having had undiagnosed Lyme for many years. After getting diagnosed and treated, she experienced some improvements, but the level of her disability was such that she would never function as she did in her life previously. She was a well-respected professional, gainfully and successfully employed, who ultimately lost her job and had to go on disability due to her illness. Even after treatment, her cognitive capacities were compromised and her physical limitations were such that she not only couldn't return to her previous job, but she was unable to return to her career. In short, she could no longer do what she was so good at when she was well.

Not surprisingly, this led to a fairly precipitous downward spiral in her mood and overall functioning. She was racked with depression and anxiety, living in constant fear of failing and thus never really trying to do anything to make her life better. In the context of her disability, she was fairly functional. She could live on her own, drive, and take care of herself. She was simply limited in how much work she could do.

When she came to me, she was essentially spending all of her time in bed with the covers pulled over her head, more or less paralyzed by the world. The only thing that got her out of the house was taking care of her mother. Megan found meaning in this and ended up volunteering then working at a nursing home. The next thing she knew she was working a few days a week, getting out of the house on a regular basis, socializing with her co-workers, making friends, and all in all, just re-engaging in life. She was not home in bed with the covers pulled over her head, expending endless energy on avoiding her fear. Instead, she engaged in what mattered, and that made all the difference.

Was her work the same as it was prior to her Lyme? No. Did it pay the same? No. Was she earning enough to get off disability and support herself? No. Did it cure her residual symptoms and lead to a Lyme-free life? No. Was her life better for having committed to an action that was in line with her values of caring for others who needed care? Unequivocally, yes. Did she need to open herself to the fear, anxiety, and pain of possible failure to take that action and eventually reap its rewards? Unequivocally, yes. We identified her value of being needed and feeling useful, did some research, and made a phone call. She stepped into her fear and came out the other side with a richer, more meaningful existence. I think you get the picture here—embrace what you can, even if it's not everything you want. It will lead to a better life.

The Tradition of Behavior Therapy

I've made a pretty big deal out of the fact that ACT is fundamentally rooted in radical Behaviorism, and there's a good reason for this. I don't plan on getting too dry and academic here, but I think it's worthwhile to know a little bit of the tradition of Behaviorism to shed some light on the solid rationale for using behavior as a treatment for behavior problems. Lyme, of course, is not a behavior problem in and of itself. But it can, like any life circumstance, lead to problematic behaviors. This is what ACT and other forms of behavioral treatments aim to address.

If you look across the realm of various common psychiatric diagnoses, almost all of them could be viewed from a behavioral perspective. Even something like an anxiety disorder, which is clearly a difficulty with emotion, is most successfully treated with behavioral approaches. If a person avoids driving on the highway because they have panic attacks when they drive on the highway, successful treatment of that panic disorder will eventually involve the person driving on the highway and learning how to experience a panic attack in such a way that it doesn't dominate their experience of driving. If the person never engages in this, then how can you say treatment has been successful?

For people who have Obsessive-Compulsive Disorder, which is characterized by repetitive, disturbing, intrusive thoughts followed by compulsive behaviors to reduce the emotional disturbance, behavioral treatments are the gold standard. If a person is compelled to wash their hands excessively after touching a doorknob triggers thoughts of being contaminated, eventually that person will have to touch the doorknob, have the intrusive thought, and experience the anxiety without washing their hands in order to be functional in the world.

There are scientifically documented successful behavioral treatments for almost all forms of human suffering. The reason I highlight this is simply so you know that ACT, and more specifically the committed action process, does not simply come from nowhere. It is deeply rooted in the science of psychology and human behavior. Those roots are far too deep and complex to go into here, but please refer to the suggested reading list if you're interested in learning more about this aspect of ACT.

Conclusions

Thus concludes our trip through the six core processes of ACT that are designed to help you increase your psychological flexibility and lead to a more meaningful, enriched, and fuller life. You may have noticed as we moved into each new process that the previous processes would occasionally come back into the picture. That was especially the case for committed action, which serves as a nice transition into the final chapter where we'll tie all of the processes together to gain a real understanding of the fluid nature of the model.

Chapter 9

Bringing It All Together

All is connected...no one thing can change by itself.
Paul Hawken

Some Final Thoughts

Now that you know all of the pieces of ACT, it's time to see how connected and fluid the model is and how each process relates to one another. What's great about ACT is that if you ever find yourself stuck—in life or just on a particular process in ACT—you can actually get yourself "unstuck" and more psychologically flexible through engaging with *any other ACT process*. Rigidity is the enemy of ACT and thus the enemy of your well-being. So let's take a moment to review the model and then put it all together.

The Hexaflex Revisited

If you recall, way back in Chapter 2, I introduced you to a weird-looking, complex diagram that illustrated the ACT model. You might have been a bit overwhelmed by that back then, but hopefully you're feeling more comfortable with it now. Take another look at the diagram and see if you notice anything important.

As you can see, the six core processes are all contributing factors to developing psychological flexibility or "the ability to contact the present moment more fully as a conscious human being, and to change or persist in behavior when doing so serves valued ends" (Hayes et al, 2012). Each of the core processes flows into and contributes to psychological flexibility.

You will also notice that each process is connected to every other process in the model. I can't emphasize enough

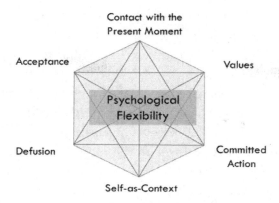

Figure 9.1: The Hexaflex Model of Psychological Flexibility
(reprinted with permission from Hayes et al, 2012)

how important this is. Above all, ACT is fluid and flexible. Remembering this will help you immensely on your journey through life and in coping with your illness.

As clinicians, we're trained in ACT to enhance each core process by not only working on that process, but by *coming at it through the other processes*. You may have noticed that there's a certain degree of overlap in the model. For example, when you learned about defusion and worked on that skill then moved to self-as-context, you may have connected the two and realized that self-as-context is essentially a defusion process, just applied to the self instead of individual thoughts. Likewise, it's very difficult to be fully present in the moment if you're not also tapping into some level of acceptance. It's nearly impossible to engage in committed action if you have not done good values work. If you look really closely at any of the core processes, you can see that they are intimately connected to every other process.

This is very useful information to have because when you get stuck—and you will get stuck, because we all do—rather than hammering away at just one process, you can actually enhance your ability to engage in it by tapping into another one that you may feel more connected to at that moment. For example, let's say you are having a lot of difficulty accepting the anxiety that often comes with medical appointments. You might do the "Take a Ride on a Balloon" or "Giving It Form" exercises from Chapter 4, but for some reason it just isn't hitting home the way you'd like. You may be struggling mightily with those feelings, being pulled hard to escape or control the anxiety, cancel the appointment, or just go through the motions and not have the honest but hard conversation with your doctor because you're afraid of what the outcome might be. Rather than continuing to do what doesn't seem to be working, you can go in a few different directions here.

If you do some values work to reinforce how important your health is to you and your family, friends, and loved ones, you may be able to connect with those values and see that committed actions towards them is essential. You can recognize that the appointment is in the future and decide to focus more on your present by using an anchor—connecting with a loved one, doing a mindfulness exercise, or focusing on your senses. You can decide to shine the light from your lighthouse on the current version of yourself rather than allowing your history or self-stories to define your present self. You can use one of the defusion exercises to tap into your observing mind and get some distance between you and those uncomfortable thoughts. Any of these approaches may bring you to a better place with your level of acceptance regarding your anxiety. You have just enhanced your ability to accept discomfort in your life by focusing on values, committed action, self-as-context, or contact with the present moment. Some of these processes are on the opposite side of the model! In other words, everything about how ACT approaches psychological flexibility is multidirectional, not linear. You do not always have to open up (defuse, accept) in order to engage (values, committed action). Sometimes you can use engagement as a way to open up.

Similarly, being present in the moment almost always requires some sort of defusion or acceptance, and acceptance and defusion necessitate some sense of being present in the moment. If you're struggling with one, try coming at it from the other. Being stuck on one process doesn't mean that you can't move forward in another, which may be more helpful than you anticipated. In other words, the ACT approach is not A then B then C then D—it's much more fluid and interactive. Yes, the chapters in this book follow an order, but that order doesn't have to dictate your process. Do what works when it works. It doesn't make sense to do it any other way.

Isolation Is the Enemy, Connection Is the Cure

The fluidity of the model means that no ACT process occurs in isolation from the other processes. They are connected to one another, not just in the diagram but in your life. While you can and should work on each skill individually, as you practice more and more you'll come to realize that working each process in isolation, while better than not working a process at all, is not as effective as working them as part of a connected whole. Because each process is connected to the others, your ability to move flexibly between them will greatly enhance your psychological flexibility and hence increase the richness and quality of your life.

The same holds true in our social relationships. There's a mountain of scientific research that consistently highlights the impact of social relationships on our quality of life. Generally, the more connected we are (we're talking quality here, not necessarily quantity), the healthier we are—physically, emotionally, psychologically, and spiritually. The more isolated we are, the worse we tend to fare. In the same way you don't want to address the core processes of ACT in isolation but rather in their connectedness, you also want to be connected to others in your life. Isolation will make everything harder, and coping with Lyme is hard enough.

I mention this because Lyme, and any illness really, has a tendency to be isolating. It can affect you in a way that's not in line with who you are—you may be irritable, less interactive, less engaged, or have less energy. It can be very difficult for those who love you to see you suffering and in pain. In order to protect themselves, they may start to distance themselves from you because your pain is hard for them to deal with. Remember, you're not the only one who may try to avoid uncomfortable thoughts and feelings. Your family members may feel resentment that they have to carry more of the responsibilities in the home. You may feel guilty about not being able to do what you used to do and that your illness is making the lives of your family and those around you at best less enjoyable and at worst more difficult.

All of these factors and many more can contribute to isolation, and that lack of connection with people can take a significant toll. Reaching out for that connection may be met with a variety of responses, and some of them might be downright hurtful. None of this is anyone's fault. Lyme disease infects the entire family, even if the bacteria are not invading every family member's body.

However, you have the opportunity to approach your life and your Lyme disease from a place of psychological flexibility. If you're able to integrate the ACT model into your life and your illness, it may dramatically impact these dynamics and increase the likelihood that you're able to maintain healthy relationships and even make new ones. I would encourage all of your family members or anyone close to you to read this book as well, so you can work with one another to be more flexible and stay connected during these very difficult times. If you have a hard time reading due to your Lyme, then have someone read to you. This can be a great way to stay connected and let the people who love you help.

The bottom line is that in the ACT model and in life, isolation is the enemy. Look for the connections and the flexibility in the model to help you better engage with it in your life, and look for the same in your relationships. You will reap the rewards in ways that might surprise you.

Future Directions

As I mentioned in the Introduction, this book has been and will continue to be a bit of an experiment. In many respects, I hesitated to write it because, although ACT is a scientifically solid model, it has never been rigorously scientifically tested with people who are suffering from Lyme or other tick-borne diseases. I am a scientist at heart, and given my druthers I would have done 5–10 years of clinical trials testing the model and then written this book with full confidence that I had good scientific support for the effectiveness of using ACT to cope with Lyme.

However, I decided to take a different approach and treat this book as more of an introduction rather than a final statement. The work of the clinical trials is ahead of me, but it was my sense that people suffering with Lyme needed to get the information about ACT in their hands sooner rather than later. I view the current state of Lyme and tick-borne diseases, both in terms of their prevalence and the medical schism that exists regarding their diagnosis and treatment, as nothing less than a national public health crisis. I fear it may get worse before it gets better. I have seen far too many people suffering from this horrible illness with no real way to cope. My awareness of Lyme and my exposure to ACT coincided with one another to a point where the light bulb went off and I felt compelled to "make the introduction." I believe people suffering from Lyme need ACT and that ACT has a lot to offer people suffering from Lyme and other chronic illnesses.

This book serves as that introduction, but it's just that, the beginning of a relationship. I strongly believe much more work needs to be done investigating the effectiveness of an ACT approach with people who are suffering from Lyme. My own clinical experience and instincts tell me that it can be a powerful intervention, but I am only one clinician with a limited number of clients. I need help in getting a large research initiative off the ground—help from you, from other Lyme clinicians, and from other ACT clinicians. That's why I asked you at the end of the Introduction to go online and complete those questionnaires and why I am asking you to do them again after you've experienced the book. This data will support future work to build evidence that ACT is a viable approach to help people suffering from Lyme and other chronic illnesses to lead richer, fuller, more meaningful lives—to show that ACT can make sure your illness doesn't define who you are or the terms of your life. The science is important to me, and this book is just the beginning.

My Hope for You

It is my sincere hope that this book has been and will continue to be of some help to you. I have mixed relationships with self-help books and never thought I would find myself writing one, but the confluence of circumstances amounted to a sort of calling for me. If you have Lyme, or know anyone who does, you know that the impact of the disease is beyond severe. The physical symptoms—joint and muscle pain, fatigue, shortness of breath—are the most obvious, but not always. The emotional impact—depression, anxiety, mood swings, cognitive difficulties—can be just as debilitating, if not more so. Add in the devastation to your family, your relationships, your career, and it can seem like a different life. What many people fail to recognize is that emotionally and spiritually Lyme can make you feel like you're being turned inside out, like you are a completely different person. *You are not.* I wrote this book because I simply couldn't let that stand. I couldn't let an illness rob you of so much of who you are. I couldn't *do nothing* when I believed there was *something*

I *could* do. I believe that ACT could help you reclaim your life—your very identity—from an awful disease. So, in keeping with ACT, I acted. What you've read has been the product of that calling, and I hope that some aspect of it has positively impacted or will positively impact your life.

Lyme is a terrible illness, and it's impossible for me to wipe it out of your life. I don't possess the skill set to do that. If you can find someone who does, then by all means avail yourself of their services. In the meantime, however, you're left to cope with the impact of this illness on your life, the lives of your family, and the lives of your friends. It is in this realm that I think this book and the ACT approach can be helpful to you. Moreover, should you be so blessed as to put Lyme behind you, ACT will still be something you can carry with you. It's more than a system for coping with an awful disease; it's a way to approach your life.

If anything I've written on these pages has resonated with you, I strongly encourage you to seek out other ACT resources. There are many out there, produced by people far more steeped and knowledgeable in ACT than I am. Learning more from them will be to your benefit. Also, please feel free to educate others about Lyme, ACT, and your experience with your life, your illness, and your trials and tribulations. Precious few clinicians have an awareness of just how severe Lyme can be, how it can affect the nervous system and hence psychological functioning. If you feel up to it and it's of value to you, tell your story.

It is, after all, our connections with one another that will lead to all of us rising above human suffering.

From the Author

Thank you for purchasing *Living Beyond Lyme*. My sincere hope is that you derived as much from reading this book as I have in creating it. If you have a few moments, please feel free to add your review of the book at your favorite online site for feedback. If you were able to complete the research surveys prior to reading the book, please take a moment to visit the website and complete them again now that you've finished. Also, if you would like to connect with others who are Living Beyond Lyme, please go to: http://livingbeyondlyme.com and support one another.

Sincerely, Joseph J. Trunzo

Further Reading

Lyme Disease Resources (from various perspectives, in alphabetical order)

Websites
American Lyme Disease Foundation: www.aldf.com
Global Lyme Alliance: www.globallymealliance.org
Infectious Diseases Society of America (IDSA): www.idsociety.org
International Lyme and Associated Diseases Society (ILADS): www.ilads.org
Lyme Disease Association: www.lymediseaseassociation.org
Lymedisease.org—Advocacy, Education, & Research: www.lymedisease.org

Books
A Cure Unknown: Inside the Lyme Epidemic, by Pamela Weintraub
Lyme Madness: Rescuing My Son Down the Rabbit Hole of Chronic Lyme Disease, by Lori Dennis
The Beginner's Guide to Lyme Disease: Diagnosis and Treatment Made Simple, by Nicola McFadzean & Joseph Burrascano Jr.
When Your Child Has Lyme Disease: A Parent's Survival Guide, by Sandra K. Berenbaum & Dorothy Kupcha Leland
Why Can't I Get Better? Solving the Mystery of Lyme and Chronic Disease, by Richard Horowitz

ACT Resources

Websites
Association for Contextual Behavioral Science (ACBS): www.contextualscience.org
Kelly Wilson's website: www.onelifellc.com

Russ Harris's website for professionals and laypeople: www.actmindfully.com.au

Steve Hayes' website: www.stevenhayes.com

Books (for laypeople)

Acceptance and Commitment Therapy for Chronic Pain, by JoAnne C. Dahl, Kelly G. Wilson, Carmen Luciano, and Steven C. Hayes

Full Catastrophe Living (Revised Edition): Using the Wisdom of Your Body and Mind to Face Stress, Pain, and Illness, by Jon Kabat-Zinn

Get Out of Your Mind and Into Your Life: The New Acceptance and Commitment Therapy, by Steven C. Hayes & Spencer Smith

Happiness Trap: How to Stop Struggling & Start Living: A Guide to ACT, by Russ Harris

Things Might Go Terribly, Horribly Wrong: A Guide to Life Liberated From Anxiety, by Kelly G. Wilson & Troy Dufrene

Wherever You Go, There You Are: Mindfulness Meditation in Everyday Life, by Jon Kabat-Zinn

Books (for professionals)

Acceptance and Commitment Therapy: The Process and Practice of Mindful Change, 2nd ed., by Steven C. Hayes, Kirk D. Strosahl, & Kelly G. Wilson

ACT Made Simple: An Easy to Read Primer on Acceptance and Commitment Therapy, by Russ Harris

Mindfulness and Acceptance in Behavioral Medicine: Current Theory and Practice, edited by Lance M. McCracken

Bibliography

Chapter 1

Berghoff, W. (2012). Chronic Lyme disease and co-infections: differential diagnosis. *The Open Neurology Journal, 6*, 158–78. Date of Electronic Publication: 2012 Dec 28.

Bransfield, R. C. (2012). The psychoimmunology of Lyme/tick-borne diseases and its association with neuropsychiatric symptoms. *The Open Neurology Journal, 6*, 88–93. Date of Electronic Publication: 2012 Oct 05.

Burdash, N. and Fernandes, J. (1991). Lyme borreliosis: detecting the great imitator. *The Journal of the American Osteopathic Association, 91(6)*, 573–4, 577–8.

Burgdorfer, W. (1993). How the discovery of Borrelia burgdorferi came about. *Clinics in Dermatology, 11(3)*, 335–8.

Cameron, D. J., Johnson, L. B., and Maloney, E. L. (2014). Evidence assessments and guideline recommendations in Lyme disease: the clinical management of known tick bites, erythema migrans rashes and persistent disease. *Expert Review of Anti-infective Therapy, 12(9)*.

Centers for Disease Control (2015). https://www.cdc.gov/lyme/stats/humancases.html (retrieved January 17, 2016).

Columbia University Medical Center (2014). Lyme and Tick Borne Diseases Research Center. http://www.columbia-lyme.org/patients/controversies.html.

Companion Vector Borne Diseases (2013). http://www.cvbd.org/en/occurrence-maps/world-map (retrieved February 11, 2017).

Embers, M. E., Grasperge, B. J., Jacobs, M. B., and Philipp, M. T. (2013). Feeding of ticks on animals for transmission and xenodiagnosis in Lyme disease research. *Journal of Visualized Experiments: Jove, (78)*. Date of Electronic Publication: 2013 Aug 31.

Fallon, B. A., Nields, J. A., Parsons, B., Liebowitz, M. R., Klein, D.

F. (1993). Psychiatric manifestations of Lyme borreliosis. *The Journal of Clinical Psychiatry, 54(7)*, 263–8.
Fallon, B. A., Schwartzberg, M., Bransfield, R., Zimmerman, B., Scotti, A., Weber, C. A., and Liebowitz, M. R. (1995). Late-stage neuropsychiatric Lyme borreliosis: differential diagnosis and treatment. *Psychosomatics: Journal of Consultation Liaison Psychiatry, 36(3)*, 295–300.
Horowitz, R. (2013). *Why Can't I Get Better? Solving the Mystery of Lyme and Chronic Disease.* St. Martin Press: New York, NY.
Infectious Disease News (June 2008). https://www.healio.com/infectious-disease/emerging-diseases/news/print/infectious-disease-news/%7Bf1c3a406-74b4-4261-9c88-bbb3ac200623%7D/connecticut-attorney-general-idsa-settlelyme-disease-case (retrieved July 27, 2017).
International Lyme and Associated Diseases Society. http://www.ilads.org/lyme/lyme-quickfacts.php (retrieved February 11, 2017).
Lyme Disease Association (2013). https://www.lymediseaseassociation.org/about-lyme/cases-stats-maps-a-graphs/940-lyme-in-more-than-80-countries-worldwide (retrieved February 11, 2017).
Magnarelli, L. A. and Anderson, J. F. (1988). Ticks and biting insects infected with the etiologic agent of Lyme disease, Borrelia burgdorferi. *Journal of Clinical Microbiology, 26(8)*, 1482–6.
Pachner, A. R. (1989). Neurologic manifestations of Lyme disease, the new "great imitator". *Reviews of Infectious Diseases, 11* Suppl 6, S1482–6.
Piesman, J. and Happ, C. M. (1997). Ability of the Lyme disease spirochete Borrelia burgdorferi to infect rodents and three species of human-biting ticks (blacklegged tick, American dog tick, lone star tick) (Acari: Ixodidae). *Journal of Medical Entomology, 34(4)*, 451–6.
Stechenberg, B. W. (1988). Lyme disease: the latest great imitator.

The Pediatric Infectious Disease Journal, 7(6), 402–9.
World Health Organization and European Centre for Disease Control (2014). http://ecdc.europa.eu/en/healthtopics/vectors/world-health-day-2014/documents/factsheet-lyme-borreliosis.pdf (retrieved February 11, 2017).
Wormser, G. P., Dattwyler, R. J., Shapiro, E. D., Halperin, J. J., Steere, A. C., Klempner, M. S., et al (2006). The clinical assessment, treatment, and prevention of Lyme disease, human granulocytic anaplasmosis, and babesiosis: clinical practice guidelines by the Infectious Diseases Society of America. *Clinical Infectious Diseases, 43(9)*, 1089–134.

Chapter 2

Beck, J. S. and Beck, A. T. (2011). *Cognitive Therapy: Basics and Beyond*, 2nd ed. Guilford Press: New York, NY.
Biglan, A., and Hayes, S. C. (1996). Should the behavioral sciences become more pragmatic? The case for functional contextualism in research on human behavior. *Applied and Preventive Psychology, 5 (1)*, 47–57.
Freud, S. (1995). *The Basic Writings of Sigmund Freud: Psychopathology of Everyday Life, The Interpretation of Dreams, and Three Contributions to the Theory of Sex*. Random House: New York, NY.
Hayes, S. C., Barnes-Holmes, D., and Roche, B. (2001). *Relational Frame Theory: A Post-Skinnerian Account of Human Language and Cognition*. Klewer Academic/Plenum Publishers: New York, NY.
Hayes, S. C., Levin, M. E., Plumb-Vilardaga, J., Villatte, J. L., and Pistorello, J. (2013). Acceptance and commitment therapy and contextual behavioral science: examining the progress of a distinctive model of behavioral and cognitive therapy. *Behavior Therapy, 44 (2)*, 180–98.
Hayes, S. C., Strosahl, K. D., and Wilson, K. G. (2012). *Acceptance and Commitment Therapy: The Process and Practice of Mindful*

Change, 2nd ed. Guilford Press: New York, NY.
Hayes, S. C. and Smith, S. (2005). *Get Out of Your Mind and Into Your Life: The New Acceptance and Commitment Therapy.* New Harbinger: Oakland, CA.
Mitchell, S. A. and Black, M. J. (1996). *Freud and Beyond: A History of Modern Psychoanalytic Thought.* Basic Books: New York, NY.
Skinner, B. F. (1965). *Science and Human Behavior.* Free Press: New York, NY.
Skinner, B. F. (1976). *About Behaviorism.* Vintage: New York, NY.
Szasz, T. and Kraus, K. (1990). *Anti-Freud: Karl Kraus's Criticism of Psychoanalysis and Psychiatry.* Syracuse University Press: Syracuse, NY.
Williams, J. M. G. and Kabat-Zinn, J. (2013). *Mindfulness: Diverse Perspectives on Its Meaning, Origins and Applications.* Routledge: New York, NY.

Chapter 3

Harris, R. (2009). *ACT Made Simple: An Easy to Read Primer on Acceptance and Commitment Therapy.* New Harbinger: Oakland, CA.
Hayes, S. C., Strosahl, K., and Wilson, K. G. (1999). *Acceptance and Commitment Therapy: An Experiential Approach to Behavior Change.* Guilford Press: New York, NY.
Hayes, S. C., Strosahl, K. D., and Wilson, K. G. (2012). *Acceptance and Commitment Therapy: The Process and Practice of Mindful Change.* 2nd ed., Guilford Press: New York, NY.
Stoddard, J. A. and Afari, N. (2014). *The Big Book of ACT Metaphors.* New Harbinger: Oakland, CA.
Titchener, E. B. (1916). *A Beginner's Guide to Psychology.* Macmillan: New York, NY.
Wilson, K. G. and DuFrene, T. (2010). *Things Might Go Terribly, Horribly Wrong: A Guide to Life Liberated from Anxiety.* New Harbinger: Oakland, CA.

Chapter 4

Bricker, J. B. (2011). Acceptance and commitment therapy: A promising approach to smoking cessation. In, McCracken, L. M. (Ed.), *Mindfulness and Acceptance in Behavioral Medicine: Current Theory and Practice* (pp. 107–30). New Harbinger: Oakland, CA.

Carlson, L. E. and Halifax, J. (2011). Mindfulness for cancer and terminal illness. In, McCracken, L. M. (Ed.), *Mindfulness and Acceptance in Behavioral Medicine: Current Theory and Practice* (pp. 159–83). New Harbinger: Oakland, CA.

Dahl, J. and Lundgren, T. (2011). Analysis and treatment of epilepsy using mindfulness, acceptance, values, and countermeasures. In, McCracken, L. M. (Ed.), *Mindfulness and Acceptance in Behavioral Medicine: Current Theory and Practice* (pp. 61–78). New Harbinger: Oakland, CA.

Dahl, J., Wilson, K. G., Luciano, C. and Hayes, S. C. (2005). *Acceptance and Commitment Therapy for Chronic Pain*. Context Press: Reno, NV.

Frankl, Viktor (2006). *Man's Search for Meaning*. Beacon Press: Boston, MA.

Gregg, J. A., Almada, P. and Schmidt, E. (2011). Health behavior problems in diabetes, obesity, and secondary prevention. In, McCracken, L. M. (Ed.), *Mindfulness and Acceptance in Behavioral Medicine: Current Theory and Practice* (pp. 79–106). New Harbinger: Oakland, CA.

Harris, R. (2009). *ACT Made Simple: An Easy to Read Primer on Acceptance and Commitment Therapy*. New Harbinger: Oakland, CA.

Hayes, S. C., Strosahl, K. D., and Wilson, K. G. (1999) *Acceptance and Commitment Therapy: An Experiential Approach to Behavior Change*. Guilford Press: New York, NY.

Hayes, S. C., Strosahl, K. D., and Wilson, K. G. (2012). *Acceptance and Commitment Therapy: The Process and Practice of Mindful Change*. 2nd ed., Guilford Press: New York, NY.

Henwood, P. and Ellis, J. A. (2004). Chronic neuropathic pain in spinal cord injury: the patient's perspective. *Pain Research and Management, 9(1),* 39–45.

Lundh, L. G. (2011). Insomnia. In, McCracken, L. M. (Ed.), *Mindfulness and Acceptance in Behavioral Medicine: Current Theory and Practice* (pp. 131–58). New Harbinger: Oakland, CA.

Summers, J. D., Rapoff, M. A., Varghese, G., Porter, K., and Palmer, R. E. (1991). Psychosocial factors in chronic spinal cord injury pain. *Pain, 47(2),* 183–9.

Vowles, K. E. and Thompson, M. (2011). Acceptance and commitment therapy for chronic pain. In, McCracken, L. M. (Ed.), *Mindfulness and Acceptance in Behavioral Medicine: Current Theory and Practice* (pp. 31–60). New Harbinger: Oakland, CA.

Weitzner, E., Surca, S., Wiese, S., Dion, A., Renwick, R. and Yoshida, K. (2011). Getting on with life: positive experiences of living with a spinal cord injury. *Qualitative Health Research, 21(11),* 1455–68.

Wilson, K. G. and DuFrene, T. (2010). *Things Might Go Terribly, Horribly Wrong: A Guide to Life Liberated from Anxiety.* New Harbinger: Oakland, CA.

Chapter 5

Harris, R. (2009). *ACT Made Simple: An Easy to Read Primer on Acceptance and Commitment Therapy.* New Harbinger: Oakland, CA.

Hayes, S. C., Strosahl, K., and Wilson, K. G. (1999). *Acceptance and Commitment Therapy: An Experiential Approach to Behavior Change.* Guilford Press: New York, NY.

Pakenham, K. and Fleming, M., (2011). Relations between acceptance of multiple sclerosis and positive and negative adjustments. *Psychology and Health, 26(10),* 1292–309.

Scott, W., Hann, K. E. J., and McCracken, L. M. (2016). A

comprehensive examination of changes in psychological flexibility following acceptance and commitment therapy for chronic pain. *Journal of Contemporary Psychotherapy, 46(3)*, 139–48.

Chapter 7
Harris, R. (2009). *ACT Made Simple: An Easy to Read Primer on Acceptance and Commitment Therapy*. New Harbinger: Oakland, CA.

Wilson, K. G. and DuFrene, T. (2010). *Things Might Go Terribly, Horribly Wrong: A Guide to Life Liberated from Anxiety*. New Harbinger: Oakland, CA.

Chapters 8 and 9
Hayes, S. C., Strosahl, K. D., and Wilson, K. G. (2012). *Acceptance and Commitment Therapy: The Process and Practice of Mindful Change*, 2nd ed. Guilford Press: New York, NY.

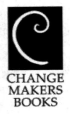

Changemakers Books

TRANSFORMATION

Transform your life, transform your world - Changemakers Books publishes for individuals committed to transforming their lives and transforming the world. Our readers seek to become positive, powerful agents of change. Changemakers Books inform, inspire, and provide practical wisdom and skills to empower us to write the next chapter of humanity's future.

If you have enjoyed this book, why not tell other readers by posting a review on your preferred book site.

Recent bestsellers from Changemakers Books are:

Integration
The Power of Being Co-Active in Work and Life
Ann Betz, Karen Kimsey-House
Integration examines how we came to be polarized in our dealing with self and other, and what we can do to move from an either/or state to a more effective and fulfilling way of being.
Paperback: 978-1-78279-865-1 ebook: 978-1-78279-866-8

Bleating Hearts
The Hidden World of Animal Suffering
Mark Hawthorne
An investigation of how animals are exploited for entertainment, apparel, research, military weapons, sport, art, religion, food, and more.
Paperback: 978-1-78099-851-0 ebook: 978-1-78099-850-3

Lead Yourself First!
Indispensable Lessons in Business and in Life
Michelle Ray
Are you ready to become the leader of your own life? Apply simple, powerful strategies to take charge of yourself, your career, your destiny.
Paperback: 978-1-78279-703-6 ebook: 978-1-78279-702-9

Burnout to Brilliance
Strategies for Sustainable Success
Jayne Morris
Routinely running on reserves? This book helps you transform your life from burnout to brilliance with strategies for sustainable success.
Paperback: 978-1-78279-439-4 ebook: 978-1-78279-438-7

Goddess Calling
Inspirational Messages & Meditations of Sacred Feminine
Liberation Thealogy
Rev. Dr. Karen Tate
A book of messages and meditations using Goddess archetypes
and mythologies, aimed at educating and inspiring those with the
desire to incorporate a feminine face of God into their
spirituality.
Paperback: 978-1-78279-442-4 ebook: 978-1-78279-441-7

The Master Communicator's Handbook
Teresa Erickson, Tim Ward
Discover how to have the most communicative impact in this
guide by professional communicators with over 30 years of
experience advising leaders of global organizations.
Paperback: 978-1-78535-153-2 ebook: 978-1-78535-154-9

Meditation in the Wild
Buddhism's Origin in the Heart of Nature
Charles S. Fisher Ph.D.
A history of Raw Nature as the Buddha's first teacher, inspiring
some followers to retreat there in search of truth.
Paperback: 978-1-78099-692-9 ebook: 978-1-78099-691-2

Ripening Time
Inside Stories for Aging with Grace
Sherry Ruth Anderson
Ripening Time gives us an indispensable guidebook for growing
into the deep places of wisdom as we age.
Paperback: 978-1-78099-963-0 ebook: 978-1-78099-962-3

Striking at the Roots
A Practical Guide to Animal Activism
Mark Hawthorne
A manual for successful animal activism from an author with first-hand experience speaking out on behalf of animals.
Paperback: 978-1-84694-091-0 ebook: 978-1-84694-653-0

Voices of the Sacred Feminine
Conversations to Re-Shape Our World
Rev. Dr. Karen Tate
If we can envision it, we can manifest it! Discover conversations that help us begin to re-shape the world!
Paperback: 978-1-78279-510-0 ebook: 978-1-78279-509-4

Readers of ebooks can buy or view any of these bestsellers by clicking on the live link in the title. Most titles are published in paperback and as an ebook. Paperbacks are available in traditional bookshops. Both print and ebook formats are available online.

Find more titles and sign up to our readers' newsletter at
http://www.johnhuntpublishing.com/transformation
Follow us on Facebook at
https://www.facebook.com/Changemakersbooks